A PHY[...]
GUI[...]

For Elsevier:

Commissioning Editor: Rita Demetriou-Swanwick
Development Editor: Veronika Watkins
Project Manager: Gail Wright
Design Direction: Erik Bigland
Illustration Manager: Bruce Hogarth

A PHYSIOTHERAPIST'S GUIDE TO CLINICAL MEASUREMENT

John Fox MSc MCSP
*Lecturer, School of Healthcare Studies,
Cardiff University, Cardiff, UK*

Richard Day BSc(Hons)
*Lecturer, School of Healthcare Studies,
Cardiff University, Cardiff, UK*

CHURCHILL LIVINGSTONE
ELSEVIER

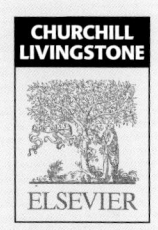

Edinburgh London New York Oxford Philadelphia
St Louis Sydney Toronto 2009

CHURCHILL
LIVINGSTONE
ELSEVIER

An imprint of Elsevier Limited

© 2009, Elsevier Limited. All rights reserved.

No part of this publication may be reproduced, stored in a retrieval system, or transmitted in any form or by any means, electronic, mechanical, photocopying, recording or otherwise, without the prior permission of the Publishers. Permissions may be sought directly from Elsevier's Health Sciences Rights Department, 1600 John F. Kennedy Boulevard, Suite 1800, Philadelphia, PA 19103-2899, USA: phone: (+1) 215 239 3804; fax: (+1) 215 239 3805; or, e-mail: *healthpermissions@elsevier.com*. You may also complete your request on-line via the Elsevier homepage (http://www.elsevier.com), by selecting 'Support and contact' and then 'Copyright and Permission'.

First published 2009

ISBN 978-0-443-06783-9

British Library Cataloguing in Publication Data
A catalogue record for this book is available from the British Library

Library of Congress Cataloging in Publication Data
A catalog record for this book is available from the Library of Congress

Notice
Neither the Publisher nor the Authors assume any responsibility for any loss or injury and/or damage to persons or property arising out of or related to any use of the material contained in this book. It is the responsibility of the treating practitioner, relying on independent expertise and knowledge of the patient, to determine the best treatment and method of application for the patient.

The Publisher

Working together to grow libraries in developing countries

www.elsevier.com | www.bookaid.org | www.sabre.org

ELSEVIER | BOOK AID International | Sabre Foundation

ELSEVIER — your source for books, journals and multimedia in the health sciences

www.elsevierhealth.com

The publisher's policy is to use paper manufactured from sustainable forests

Printed in China

Contents

Preface vi

Acknowledgements viii

Reliability and Validity of Measurement Tools ix

1 The Hip Joint	1
2 The Knee Joint	41
3 The Ankle Joint	59
4 The Shoulder Joint	89
5 The Elbow Joint	125
6 The Wrist/Carpal Joints	149
7 The Hand	173
8 The Spine	187
9 The Respiratory System	209

Appendix 1 The Visual Analogue Scale for Pain 219

Appendix 2 Summary of Studies Assessing the Reliability and Validity of Measuring Tools in Physiotherapy 220

Index 265

Preface

This book is part of *The Physiotherapist's Toolbox* series, primarily written for the undergraduate and recently qualified therapy practitioner. Students are taught and practise a myriad of measuring techniques, which may be easily forgotten the moment they leave the practical class. We have therefore produced a practical measurement book so the student or practitioner will be able to refer to the appropriate measurement skill required with ease, and gain information on the technique from the written and photographic descriptions given.

We were particularly keen to include in the publication two measurement tools we consider to be very important to both undergraduates and practitioners and which we had not previously seen in any other texts, namely the measurement of the strength of all the major muscle groups using manual muscle testing (MMT)/Oxford grading and the measurement of respiratory function using spirometry.

We have divided the book into anatomical regions, having a chapter for each of the major joints of the body, i.e. the hip joint, knee joint, ankle joint, shoulder joint, elbow joint, wrist, hand and the spine. Anatomical knowledge is paramount when performing a measurement technique, particularly surface anatomy. We have therefore begun each chapter with a review of the anatomy of the region, giving information on the bony landmarks required to be palpated, the ligaments appropriate to the joint, and the muscles producing the movements at that joint. Further anatomical information can be sought by reading anatomical texts such as *Anatomy and Human Movement* by Palastanga et al (2006) or *Gray's Anatomy for Students* by Drake et al (2009).

To supplement the teaching within the classroom, we have found peer observation to be effective at enhancing understanding. The peer observation checklist helps to structure the observation, but is equally useful as an aid to reflection. Alongside the checklist is space which can be used to record a simulated patient record and notes on the finer intricacies of the measuring technique.

We have sought out relevant papers summarizing studies on the reliability and validity of the particular measuring tool discussed. These papers have been presented in a table format and include brief descriptions of the aims, methods, measuring procedures and results. This is not intended to be a critical appraisal of the literature and thus does not give an indication of the research quality. Most of the references are from papers readily available from the university or hospital library.

Cardiff 2009

John Fox
Richard Day

REFERENCES

Drake R, Vogl AW, Mitchell AWM 2009 Gray's anatomy for students. Churchill Livingstone, Philadelphia

Palastanga N, Field D, Soames RW 2006 Anatomy and human movement: structure and function, 5th edn. Butterworth-Heinemann, Edinburgh

Acknowledgements

We wish to thank our families and colleagues, whose encouragement and support has been invaluable throughout the writing of this book.

We are extremely grateful to Anita Holmes, Nicholas Howells, Jodie Walters and Tim Sharp for their assistance in being willing subjects for the illustrations.

Lastly, we wish to thank the staff at Elsevier who have encouraged the project and dealt patiently with all our queries and concerns.

Reliability and validity of measurement tools

RELIABILITY

'Reliability refers to the fact that a test should measure exactly the same quality or attribute each time it is used' (Hicks 2004). For example, a tape measure that stretches will not give reliable results when measuring limb girth.

Intertester (interobserver) reliability assesses the reliability of a method measured by different people on the same occasion (Jordan 2000).

Intratester (intraobserver) reliability assesses the reliability of a method measured more than once by the same person (Jordan 2000). Statistics can be used to assess variations in numerical data and therefore to assess the measurement of reliability. The main statistical test used to measure the reliability of a measuring tool is the intra-class correlation coefficient (ICC). This is a numerical value, which measures the closeness of the relationship between the two variables. The closer the figure is to -1 or $+1$, the stronger the relationship.

VALIDITY

'Validity refers to the idea that a test should measure what it is intended to measure' (Hicks 2004). There are various types of validity:

Face validity indicates that the instrument appears to measure what it is meant to measure.
Content validity is determined by judging whether or not an instrument adequately measures and represents the domain of interest.
Construct validity refers to the concept that a test should assess the theory under investigation.

Criterion validity examines the extent to which a measuring instrument provides results that can be compared to a well-established gold standard of measurement. For example, the Jamar dynamometer is the gold standard for the measurement of grip strength.

GONIOMETRIC MEASUREMENT

To assess the range of motion (ROM) of a patient's peripheral joint, a clinician will generally use a universal goniometer (Fig. 1.1). This consists of a 360° or 180° protractor, which has attached a fixed (stationary) arm and a moveable arm. At the centre of the protractor is the axis, around which the moveable arm can move.

The universal goniometer comes in a number of sizes, depending on the size of the joint being measured. In Figure 1.1, a large universal goniometer is being used to measure the hip joint, whereas Figure 3.2 shows a small universal goniometer measuring ankle plantarflexion. To measure the thumb metacarpophalangeal flexion, a small hand goniometer is used (Fig. 7.3).

To measure neck range of motion, a cervical measurement system may be used (Fig. 8.7). It consists of a special head device, easily adjustable for each size of head, on to which are placed two separate inclinometers and a compass goniometer. These are positioned on the head apparatus so that neck flexion or extension, side flexion and rotation can be easily measured.

RECORDING KNEE FLEXION/EXTENSION/ HYPEREXTENSION

There is some controversy on how to record the measurement of a patient who cannot fully extend their knee and that of a patient who has a hyperextended knee. The International Knee Documentation Committee (IKDC) has proposed the following way to record knee range of motion, where three figures are filled out for flexion/zero-point/hyperextension. Knee flexion is recorded as the number of degrees measured by the goniometer, for example 105°. If the patient is unable to fully extend the knee by, for example, 20°, then this is recorded as 105/20/0. This shows the patient has a flexion contracture of 20°. If the patient has achieved 105° of flexion and 10° hyperextension of the knee, then this would be recorded as 105/0/10. If the patient has 105° of knee flexion and full extension, then this would be recorded as 105/0/0 (Hefti et al 1993).

TAPE MEASURE

A tape measure is an inexpensive but reliable tool for measuring limb girth (Fig. 1.7), joint girth (Fig. 2.3), leg length (Fig. 3.25), spinal movements (Figs 8.1 and 8.11) and chest expansion (Fig. 9.2).

THE JAMAR HAND DYNAMOMETER

To measure grip strength, a Jamar hand dynamometer may be used. It consists of a sealed hydraulic system, with a gauge calibrated in pounds or kilograms (Fig. 6.22). It is currently regarded as the gold standard for the measurement of grip strength (Mathiowetz 2002, Shechtman et al 2005).

MANUAL MUSCLE TESTING/OXFORD GRADING

Manual muscle testing continues to be the most commonly used method for recording impairment in muscle strength. It is customary to use a 0 to 5 scale for recording muscle strength (Medical Research Council 1976). The grades can be seen in Table 0.1.

Table 0.1

Oxford grading	
Grade	Definition
0	No contraction of the muscle
1	A flicker of a contraction
2	Full range of movement with gravity eliminated
3	Full range of movement against gravity and with a hold
4	Full range of movement against a minimal resistance
5	Full range of movement against a maximal resistance

RELIABILITY AND VALIDITY OF MEASUREMENT TOOLS

SPIROMETRY

Spirometry is used to assess and monitor lung function. A spirometer measures the **vital capacity (VC)**, the **forced expiratory volume in one second (FEV_1)**, the **forced vital capacity (FVC)** and the **FEV_1/FVC ratio**.

- The **vital capacity (VC)** is the largest volume measured on maximum expiration after a maximum inspiration.
- The **forced expiratory volume in one second (FEV_1)** is the volume of air expired (exhaled) in the first second after a maximal inspiration.
- The **forced vital capacity (FVC)** is the total volume of air that can be expired (exhaled) during a maximum expiration.
- The **FEV_1/FVC ratio** is the percentage of the FVC expired in one second.

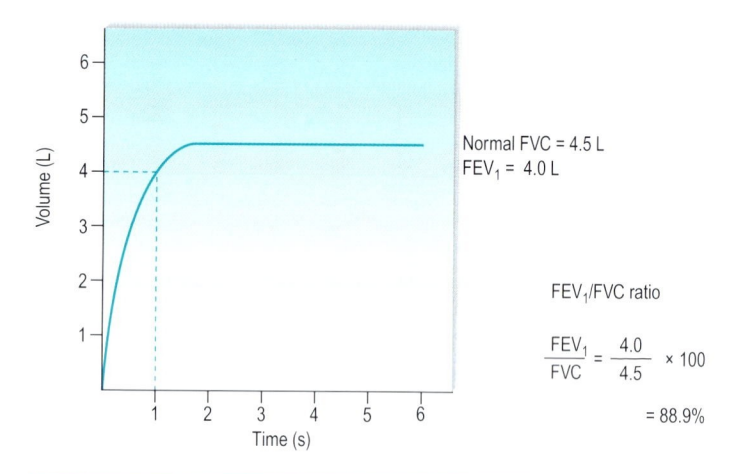

Fig 0.1 The volume–time curve in a normal patient.

Normal FVC = 4.5 L
FEV_1 = 4.0 L

FEV_1/FVC ratio

$$\frac{FEV_1}{FVC} = \frac{4.0}{4.5} \times 100 = 88.9\%$$

In an obstructive disease, such as asthma or chronic obstructive pulmonary disease (COPD), there is narrowing or obstruction of the airways.

- The volumes are normal
- Air is expired more slowly because of the obstruction of the airways
- The curve is flattened

Spirometry

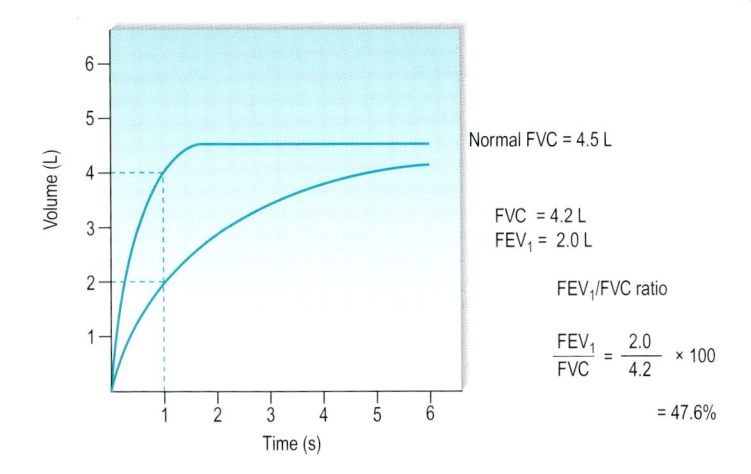

Fig 0.2 The volume–time curve in a patient with an obstructive disease.

Normal FVC = 4.5 L

FVC = 4.2 L
FEV_1 = 2.0 L

FEV_1/FVC ratio

$$\frac{FEV_1}{FVC} = \frac{2.0}{4.2} \times 100$$

= 47.6%

- The FVC is normal
- The FEV_1 is lowered
- The FEV_1/FVC ratio is lower

In a restrictive lung disease, such as pneumoconiosis, silicosis or asbestosis, there may be fibrosis or scarring of the lung.

Normal FVC = 4.5 L

FVC = 2.0 L
FEV_1 = 1.8 L

FEV_1/FVC ratio

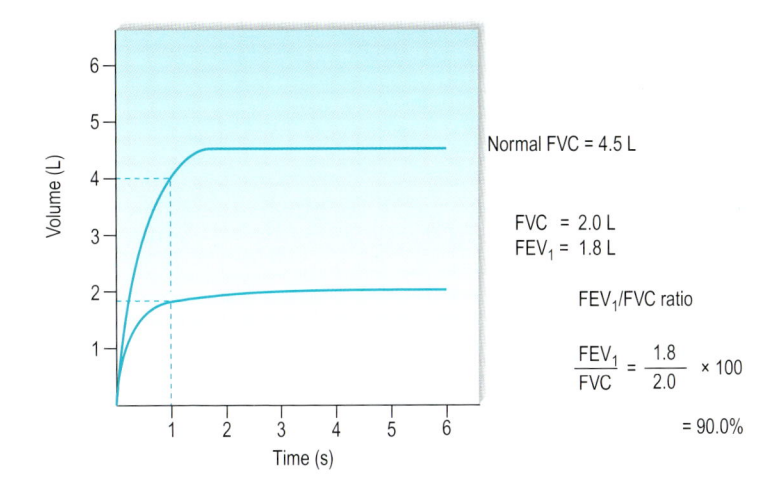

$$\frac{FEV_1}{FVC} = \frac{1.8}{2.0} \times 100$$

= 90.0%

Fig 0.3 The volume–time curve in a patient with a restrictive disease.

- The volumes are low
- The rate of emptying is normal
- The volume–time curve looks normal, but reduced
- The FVC is lowered
- The FEV_1 is lowered
- The FEV_1/FVC ratio is normal

In a combined/mixed lung disease there is a mixture of restrictive and obstructive elements.

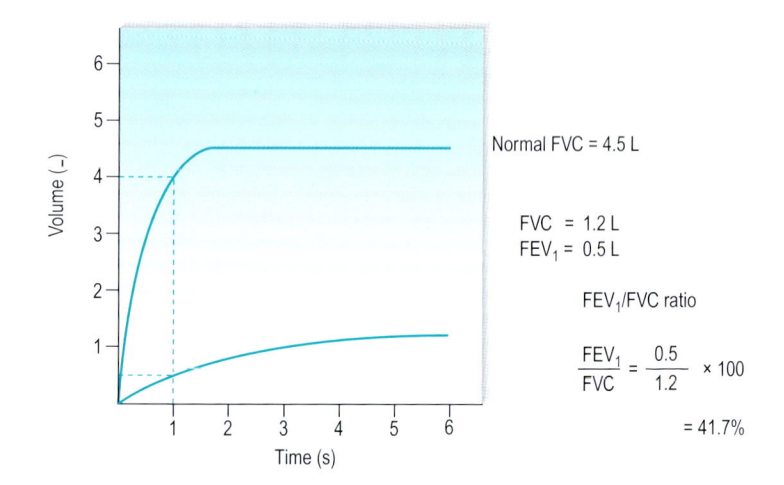

Fig 0.4 The volume–time curve in a combined/mixed patient.

- The lung volumes are reduced (restrictive)
- The airways are narrowed (obstructive)
- All parameters are affected, i.e. FVC and FEV_1 are lowered
- The FEV_1/FVC ratio is lowered

The use of a portable peak flow meter (PFM) as a tool for objectively monitoring a patient's condition is recommended in the management of asthma. The PFM measures the patient's peak expiratory flow rate (**PEFR**).

The peak expiratory flow rate (PEFR) is the greatest flow that can be sustained for 10 milliseconds on forced expiration starting from full inflation of the lungs and it is measured in litres per minute. There are several kinds of PFMs available and the Mini-Wright Peak Flow Meter is described later in the text.

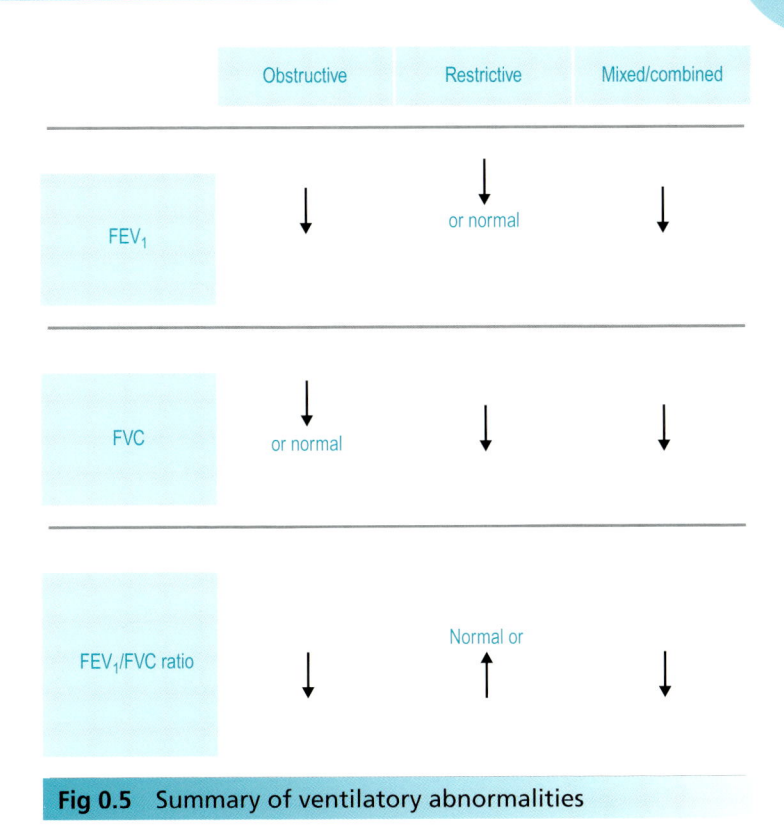

	Obstructive	Restrictive	Mixed/combined
FEV_1	↓	↓ or normal	↓
FVC	↓ or normal	↓	↓
FEV_1/FVC ratio	↓	Normal or ↑	↓

Fig 0.5 Summary of ventilatory abnormalities

REFERENCES

Hefti F, Müller W, Jakob RP, Stäubli H-U 1993 Evaluation of knee ligament injuries with the IKDC form. Knee Surgery, Sports Traumatology, Arthroscopy 1:226–234

Hicks C 2004 Research methods for clinical therapists, 4th edn. Churchill Livingstone, Edinburgh, p. 243

Jordan K 2000 Assessment of published reliability studies for cervical spine range-of-motion measurement tools. Journal of Manipulative and Physiological Therapeutics 23(3):180–195

Mathiowetz V 2002 Comparison of Rolyan and Jamar dynamometers for measuring grip strength. Occupational Therapy International 9(3):201–209

Medical Research Council 1976 Aids to the examination of the peripheral nervous system. Her Majesty's Stationery Office, London

Shechtman O, Gestewitz L, Kimble C 2005 Reliability and validity of the DynEx dynamometer. Journal of Hand Therapy 18(3): 339–347

BIBLIOGRAPHY AND FURTHER READING

Hough A 2001 Physiotherapy in respiratory care, 3rd edn. Nelson Thornes, Cheltenham

Pryor JA Prasad SA 2008 Physiotherapy for respiratory and cardiac problems: adults and paediatrics, 4th edn. Churchill Livingstone, London

CHAPTER 1

The hip joint

ANATOMY 1
  Bony landmarks to be palpated 2
  Ligaments 2
  Muscles 3
    Extensors 3
    Flexors 4
    Abductors 5
    Adductors 6
    Lateral rotators 7
    Medial rotators 8
MEASUREMENT 8
  Range of movement 9
    Extension 9
    Flexion 10
    Abduction 11
    Adduction 12
    Lateral (external) rotation 13
    Medial (internal) rotation 14
    Observational/reflective checklist 16
  Muscle bulk 17
    Limb girth: thigh 17
    Observational/reflective checklist 19
  Muscle strength: Oxford muscle grading 20
    Extensors 20
    Flexors 22
    Abductors 25
    Adductors 27
    Lateral (external) rotators 30
    Medial (internal) rotators 32
  Leg length 36
    True length of limb 38
    Site of true shortening 38
    Apparent shortening 38

ANATOMY

1. The hip joint is a synovial ball and socket joint.
2. It is an articulation between the head of the femur and the acetabulum of the innominate (hip) bone.
3. It has a strong joint capsule, attaching to the articular margins of the acetabulum and the femoral neck.

THE HIP JOINT

4. It has very strong capsular ligaments – the iliofemoral, pubofemoral and ischiofemoral ligaments.
5. The acetabular labrum deepens the acetabulum.
6. The movements that take place at the hip joint are: flexion, extension, abduction, adduction, lateral (external) rotation and medial (internal) rotation.

BONY LANDMARKS TO BE PALPATED

The innominate (hip) bone – iliac crest, anterior superior iliac spine (ASIS), posterior superior iliac spine (PSIS), pubic tubercle, ischial tuberosity.

The femur – greater trochanter.

LIGAMENTS

Table 1.1

The ligaments			
Ligament	Origin	Insertion	Limitation to movement
Iliofemoral ligament	Anterior inferior iliac spine (AIIS) of the innominate (hip) bone	Intertrochanteric line of the femur	This ligament limits hip extension, adduction and lateral rotation
Pubofemoral ligament	Iliopubic eminence and superior pubic ramus of the innominate bone	Lower part of the intertrochanteric line of the femur	This ligament limits hip extension, abduction and lateral rotation
Ischiofemoral ligament	Body of the ischium behind and below the acetabulum of the innominate bone	Superior part of the neck and root of the greater trochanter of the femur	This ligament limits hip extension, abduction and medial rotation
Transverse ligament of the acetabulum	It goes across the deficient inferior acetabular rim of the innominate bone		
Ligamentum teres	Margins of the acetabular notch of the innominate bone	Fovea capitis on the head of the femur	The ligament is taut in flexion and adduction

MUSCLES
Extensors

Table 1.2

The extensors of the hip				
Muscle	Origin	Insertion	Nerve supply	Action(s)
Gluteus maximus	Gluteal surface of the ilium, iliac crest of the innominate (hip) bone, coccyx, sacrum and sacrotuberous ligament	Gluteal tuberosity of the femur (1/4), (3/4) form the iliotibial tract	Inferior gluteal nerve L5, S1, 2	Extension of the hip, extension of the knee – through the iliotibial tract
Semitendinosus (hamstrings)	Ischial tuberosity of the innominate (hip) bone	Medial surface of medial condyle of tibia	Sciatic nerve L5, S1, 2	Extension of the hip and flexion of the knee
Semimembranosus (hamstrings)	Ischial tuberosity of the innominate (hip) bone	Posteromedial surface of medial condyle of tibia	Sciatic nerve L5, S1, 2	Extension of the hip and flexion of the knee
Biceps femoris (hamstrings)	Ischial tuberosity of the innominate (hip) bone	Head of fibula	Sciatic nerve L5, S1, 2	Extension of the hip and flexion of the knee

THE HIP JOINT

Flexors

Table 1.3

The flexors of the hip

Muscle	Origin	Insertion	Nerve supply	Action(s)
Psoas major	Transverse processes of all lumbar vertebrae, bodies of 12th thoracic and all lumbar vertebrae, and intervertebral disc above all the lumbar vertebrae	Lesser trochanter of the femur	Branches from lumbar plexus L2, 3	Flexion of the hip, flexion of the trunk
Iliacus	Upper two-thirds of iliac fossa of the innominate bone, ala of sacrum	Lesser trochanter of the femur	Femoral nerve L2, 3	Flexion of the hip
Pectineus	Superior ramus of the pubis, iliopubic eminence and pubic tubercle of the innominate bone	Pectineal line on the femur	Femoral nerve L2, 3	Flexion and adduction of the hip
Rectus femoris	Anterior inferior iliac spine (AIIS) of the innominate bone and reflected head above the acetabulum	Upper border of the patella	Femoral nerve L2, 3, 4	Flexion of the hip and extension of the knee
Sartorius	Anterior superior iliac spine (ASIS) of the innominate bone	Medial side of the body of the tibia, with gracilis and semitendinosus	Femoral nerve L2, 3	Flexion of hip and knee, lateral rotation and abduction of the thigh, and medial rotation of the tibia on the femur
Tensor fascia lata	Anterior one-third of the outer lip of the iliac crest of the innominate (hip) bone	Blends into the iliotibial tract, which in turn inserts into the lateral aspect of the patella tendon/ retinaculum	Superior gluteal nerve L4, 5	Flexion, abduction and medial rotation of the hip. Extension of the knee

Abductors

Table 1.4

The abductors of the hip				
Muscle	Origin	Insertion	Nerve supply	Action(s)
Gluteus maximus	Gluteal surface of the ilium, iliac crest of the innominate bone, coccyx, sacrum and sacrotuberous ligament	Gluteal tuberosity of the femur (1/4), (3/4) form the iliotibial tract	Inferior gluteal nerve L5, S1, 2	Extension of the hip, extension of the knee – through the iliotibial tract
Gluteus medius	Gluteal surface of the ilium, between the posterior and anterior gluteal lines of the innominate (hip) bone	Superolateral side of the greater trochanter of the femur	Superior gluteal nerve L4, 5, S1	Abduction and medial rotation of the hip
Gluteus minimus	Gluteal surface of the ilium, in front of the anterior and above the inferior gluteal lines of the innominate bone	Anterosuperior aspect of the greater trochanter of the femur	Superior gluteal nerve L4, 5, S1	Abduction and medial rotation of the hip
Tensor fascia lata	Anterior one-third of the outer lip of the iliac crest of the innominate (hip) bone	Between the two layers of the iliotibial tract	Superior gluteal nerve L4, 5	Abduction, flexion and medial rotation of the hip

Adductors

Table 1.5

The adductors of the hip				
Muscle	Origin	Insertion	Nerve supply	Action(s)
Adductor magnus	Ischial tuberosity of the innominate (hip) bone	Upper part of linea aspera and adductor tubercle of femur	Obturator nerve L2, 3	Adduction of the hip. May act as a medial or lateral rotation of the hip, depending on the position of the thigh
Adductor longus	The body of the pubis of the innominate bone	Middle half of linea aspera of femur	Obturator nerve L2, 3, 4	Adduction of the thigh
Adductor brevis	Lateral part of the body and inferior ramus of the pubis of the innominate bone	Upper half of the linea aspera of the femur	Obturator nerve L2, 3, 4	Adduction of the thigh
Gracilis	Front of the body of the pubis, inferior pubic and ischial rami of the innominate bone	Medial surface of the body of the tibia	Obturator nerve L2, 3	Adduction of the thigh and flexion of the knee
Pectineus	Superior ramus of the pubis, iliopubic eminence and pubic tubercle of the innominate bone	Pectineal line on the femur	Femoral nerve L2, 3	Flexion and adduction of the hip

Lateral rotators

Table 1.6

The lateral rotators of the hip

Muscle	Origin	Insertion	Nerve supply	Action(s)
Gluteus maximus	Gluteal surface of the ilium, iliac crest of the innominate (hip) bone, coccyx, sacrum and sacrotuberous ligament	Gluteal tuberosity of the femur (1/4), (3/4) form the iliotibial tract	Inferior gluteal nerve L5, S1, 2	Extension of the hip, extension of the knee – through the iliotibial tract
Piriformis	Front of the 2nd to 4th sacral segments, gluteal surface of the ilium of the innominate bone and sacrotuberous ligament	Upper border and medial side of greater trochanter of femur	Anterior rami of the sacral plexus L5, S1, 2	Lateral rotation of hip and abduction when the subject is in a sitting position
Obturator internus	Internal surface of the obturator membrane and surrounding bony margin of the innominate bone	Medial surface of the greater trochanter of the femur	Nerve to obturator internus L5, S1, 2	Lateral rotation of hip and abduction when the subject is in a sitting position
Gemellus superior	Gluteal surface of the ischial spine of the innominate bone	Medial surface of the greater trochanter of the femur	Medial surface of the greater trochanter of the femur	Lateral rotation of hip and abduction when the subject is in a sitting position
Gemellus inferior	Upper part of the ischial tuberosity of the innominate bone	Blends with obturator internus and attaches into the medial surface of the greater trochanter of the femur	Nerve to quadratus femoris L4, 5, S1	Lateral rotation of hip and abduction when the subject is in a sitting position

Medial rotators

Table 1.7

The medial rotators of the hip				
Muscle	Origin	Insertion	Nerve supply	Action(s)
Tensor fascia lata	Anterior one-third of the outer lip of the iliac crest of the innominate (hip) bone	Between the two layers of the iliotibial tract	Superior gluteal nerve L4, 5	Abduction, flexion and medial rotation of the hip
Gluteus medius	Gluteal surface of ilium between the posterior and anterior gluteal lines of the innominate (hip) bone	Superolateral side of the greater trochanter of the femur	Superior gluteal nerve L4, 5, S1	Abduction and medial rotation of the hip
Gluteus minimus	Gluteal surface of the ilium, in front of the anterior and above the inferior gluteal lines of the innominate (hip) bone	Anterosuperior aspect of the greater trochanter of the femur	Superior gluteal nerve L4, 5, S1	Abduction and medial rotation of the hip

MEASUREMENT

Clinical tip
Palpation. The centre of the hip joint lies in a horizontal plane, passing through the top of the greater trochanter. The joint centre lies 1 cm below the middle third of the inguinal ligament (this goes from the anterior superior iliac spine (ASIS) to the pubic tubercle).

RANGE OF MOVEMENT
Extension

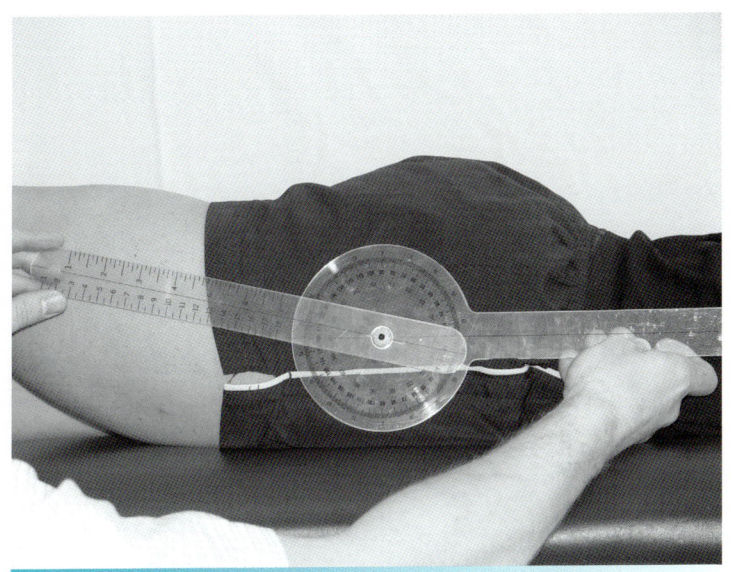

Fig 1.1 Goniometric measurement of hip extension.

Starting position: The patient is positioned in prone lying on a plinth. Their hip is in neutral and knee in extension. Their feet must be over the end of the plinth.
Goniometer axis: The axis of the goniometer is placed over the greater trochanter of the femur.
Stationary arm: This is parallel to the mid-axillary line of the trunk.
Moveable arm: This is parallel to the longitudinal axis of the femur, pointing towards the lateral epicondyle of the femur.
Command to patient: 'Lift your leg backwards as far as you can.'
End position: The hip is extended to the limit of motion.
Trick movement: Extension of the lumbar spine.

> **Clinical tip**
> The greater trochanter can be found by palpating the iliac crest – at its mid-point, one hand span down should get you to the area of the greater trochanter. You will feel movement at the greater trochanter on medial and lateral rotation of the leg.

THE HIP JOINT

Flexion

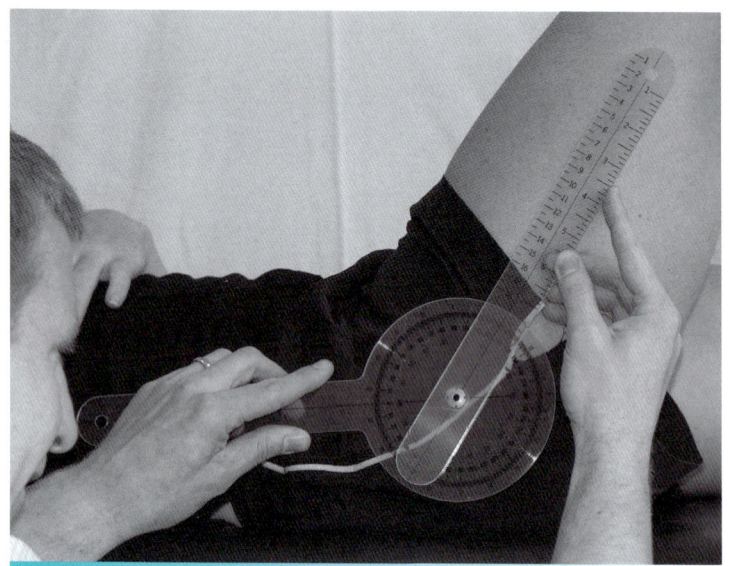

Fig 1.2 Goniometric measurement of hip flexion.

Starting position: The patient is positioned in supine lying on the plinth. Their hip is in neutral and the knee is in extension.
Goniometer axis: The goniometer axis is placed over the greater trochanter of the femur.
Stationary arm: This is parallel to the mid-axillary line of the trunk.
Moveable arm: This is parallel to the longitudinal axis of the femur, pointing towards the lateral epicondyle of the femur.
Command to patient: 'Bend your knee up towards your chest as far as you can, sliding your heel up the plinth.'
End position: The hip is flexed to the limit of motion. The heel is moved towards the buttock to the limit of hip flexion.
Trick movement: Flexion of the lumbar spine.

> NB: It may be necessary to reposition the stationary and moveable arms of the goniometer prior to taking the reading, as they may have moved when the patient flexed their hip.

Abduction

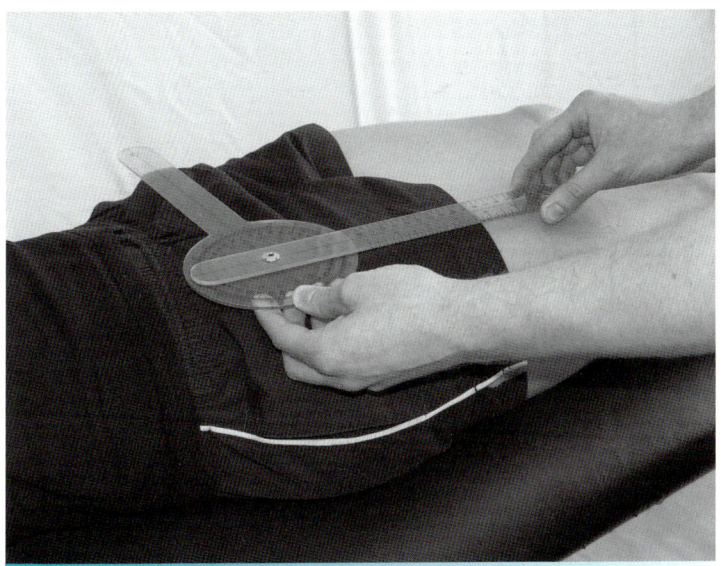

Fig 1.3 Goniometric measurement of hip abduction.

Starting position: The patient is positioned in supine lying on the plinth. Their hip is in neutral and their knee is in extension. Ensure the pelvis is level.
Goniometer axis: The goniometer axis is placed over the anterior superior iliac spine (ASIS) of the innominate bone, on the side of the hip being measured.
Stationary arm: This is placed along a line between the two ASISs.
Moveable arm: This is parallel to the longitudinal axis of the femur, pointing to the middle of the patella.
Command to patient: 'Take your leg out sideways as far as you can. Keep your great toe pointing towards the ceiling.'
End position: The hip is abducted to the limit of motion.
Trick movement: Lateral (external) rotation of the hip.

Adduction

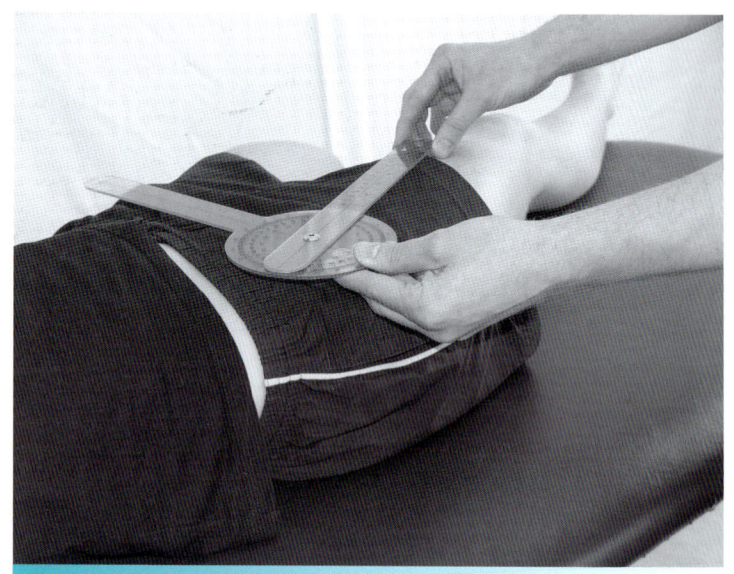

Fig 1.4 Goniometric measurement of adduction of the hip.

Starting position: The patient is positioned in supine lying on the plinth. Their hip is in neutral and their knee is in extension. Ensure the pelvis is level. The opposite leg is abducted over the side of the plinth and the foot is resting on a stool.
Goniometer axis: The goniometer axis is placed over the anterior superior iliac spine (ASIS) of the innominate bone, on the side of the hip being measured.
Stationary arm: This is placed along a line between the two ASISs.
Moveable arm: This is parallel to the longitudinal axis of the femur, pointing to the middle of the patella.
Command to patient: 'Bring your leg in towards your opposite leg as far as you can. Keep your great toe pointing towards the ceiling.'
End position: The hip is adducted to the limit of motion.
Trick movement: Medial (internal) rotation of the hip.

Lateral (external) rotation

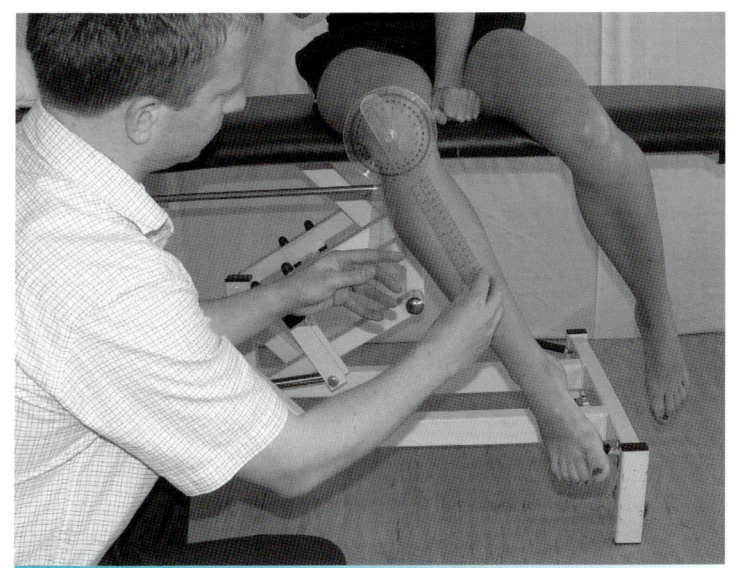

Fig 1.5 Goniometric measurement of lateral rotation of the hip.

Starting position: The patient is positioned in sitting on a raised plinth. Their hip is in 90° of flexion and neutral rotation, with the knee flexed to 90°. The opposite hip is abducted and the foot is supported on a stool.
Goniometer axis: The axis of the goniometer is placed over the mid-point of the patella.
Stationary arm: This is perpendicular to the floor.
Moveable arm: This is parallel to the anterior border of the tibia.
Command to patient: 'Turn your leg and foot in as far as you can.'
End position: The hip is laterally (externally) rotated to the limit of motion, so that the leg and foot move in a medial direction.

> *Clinical tip*
> This may seem a confusing movement: turning the foot in produces lateral (external) rotation at the hip and turning the foot out produces medial (internal) rotation. It may help if you think what would happen if a nail was inserted anteriorly into the femoral shaft – it would move laterally when the foot was turned in and medially when the foot was turned out.

Medial (internal) rotation

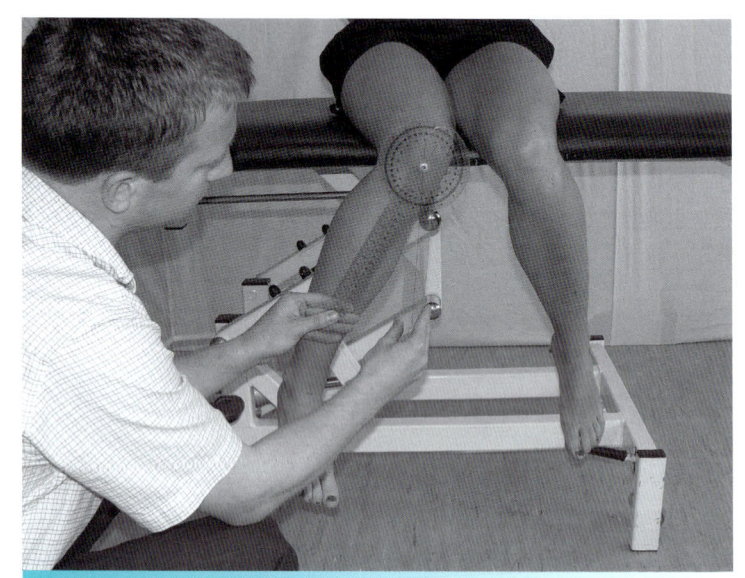

Fig 1.6 Goniometric measurement of medial rotation of the hip.

Starting position: The patient is positioned in sitting on a raised plinth. Their hip is in 90° of flexion and neutral rotation, with the knee flexed to 90°. The opposite hip is abducted and the foot is supported on a stool.
Goniometer axis: The axis of the goniometer is placed over the mid-point of the patella.
Stationary arm: This is perpendicular to the floor.
Moveable arm: This is parallel to the anterior border of the tibia.
Command to patient: 'Turn your leg and foot out as far as you can.'
End position: The hip is medially (internally) rotated to the limit of motion, so that the leg and foot move in a lateral direction.

> **Clinical tip**
> This may seem a confusing movement: turning the foot in produces lateral (external) rotation at the hip and turning the foot out produces medial (internal) rotation. It may help if you think what would happen if a nail was inserted anteriorly into the femoral shaft – it would move laterally when the foot was turned in and medially when the foot was turned out.

Measurement 15

Notes

Treatment record

THE HIP JOINT

Observational/reflective checklist

Observational/reflective checklist			
Observation		Y/N	Comments
Introduction and preparation for the skill	Was the treatment area properly prepared for the patient, e.g. pillow, blanket, safe environment, etc.?		
	Did the therapist introduce him/herself?		
	Was the patient comfortable?		
	Was the patient adequately exposed/draped?		
	Was an explanation of the procedure given?		
	Was the explanation clear and succinct?		
	Was consent obtained?		
Performing the skill	Was the plinth set at the correct height?		
	Was the therapist's posture compromised?		
	Did the therapist identify the joint and other relevant bony landmarks?		
	Was the goniometer correctly aligned?		
	Was the reading of the joint range of movement accurate?		
	Did the therapist compare both sides of the body?		
Safe and effective performance of the technique	Was the procedure carried out with due care and attention?		
How would you rate the proficiency in the overall performance of the skill?	Excellent		
	Very good		
	Good		
	Satisfactory		
	Borderline		
	Fail		

MUSCLE BULK
Limb girth: thigh

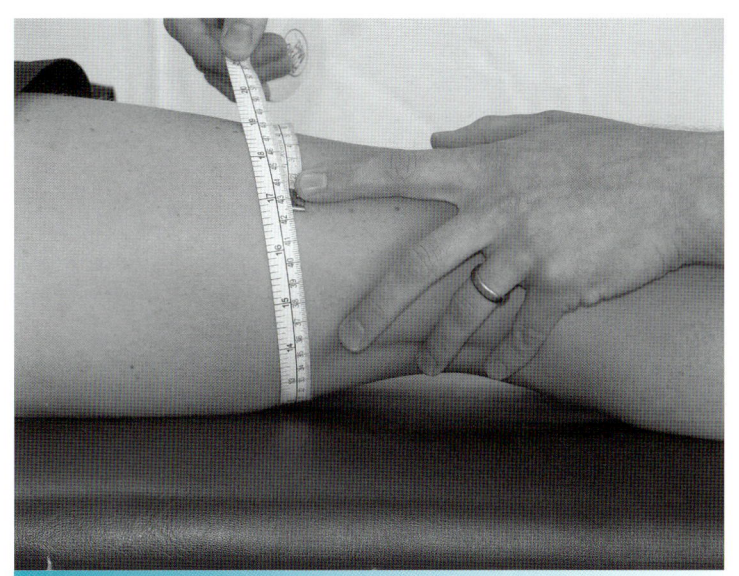

Fig 1.7 Measurement of the girth of the thigh.

Patient's position: The patient is positioned in long sitting/half lying on a plinth, well supported. The knees are in passive extension so that the thigh and calf muscles are relaxed.

Method: Three points are marked – 15 cm (6 inches), 20 cm (8 inches) and 25 cm (10 inches) from the distal end of the tibial tuberosity. The limb is encircled with a tape measure at each marked point. The circumferential measurements are then recorded.

Repeat three times and produce an average reading, then repeat the procedure on the other limb to compare the measurements.

Points to note:
  The state of the tape measure – is it stretched?
  The muscles must be relaxed.
  Keep the tape measure straight (not twisted).
  Measure consistently – at the top/bottom of the tape, and either in centimetres or in inches.

18 THE HIP JOINT

Notes

Treatment record

Measurement

Observational/reflective checklist

Observational/reflective checklist			
Observation		**Y/N**	**Comments**
Introduction and preparation for the skill	Was the treatment area properly prepared for the patient, e.g. pillow, blanket, safe environment, etc.?		
	Did the therapist introduce him/herself?		
	Was the patient comfortable?		
	Was the patient adequately exposed/draped?		
	Was an explanation of the procedure given?		
	Was the explanation clear and succinct?		
	Was consent obtained?		
Performing the skill	Was the plinth set at the correct height?		
	Was the therapist's posture compromised?		
	Did the therapist identify the joint and other relevant bony landmarks?		
	Was the tape measure correctly aligned?		
	Was the reading of the limb girth accurate?		
	Did the therapist compare both sides of the body?		
Safe and effective performance of the technique	Was the procedure carried out with due care and attention?		
How would you rate the proficiency in the overall performance of the skill?	Excellent		
	Very good		
	Good		
	Satisfactory		
	Borderline		
	Fail		

THE HIP JOINT

MUSCLE STRENGTH: OXFORD MUSCLE GRADING

Extensors

Grade 0 – 'No contraction' and Grade 1 – 'Flicker of a contraction'

Patient's position: The patient is positioned in prone lying on the plinth.

Clinician's position: The clinician is standing by the patient, with both hands palpating the gluteus maximus muscle.

Command to patient: 'Try and tighten your seat muscles.'

Clinical tip: Closely observing and feeling the muscle is essential in enabling the clinician to pick up on even the smallest flicker of a contraction.

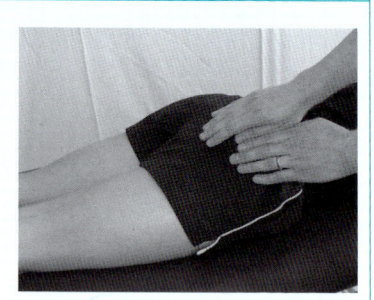

Fig 1.8 Oxford muscle grading for the hip extensors – Grades 0 and 1.

Grade 2 – 'Full range of movement (ROM) with the effects of gravity eliminated'

Patient's position: The patient is positioned in side lying on the plinth. Their leg is supported in full hip flexion.

Clinician's position: The clinician is standing behind the patient, supporting the right limb with one hand under the knee and the other supporting around the foot.

Command to the patient: 'Try and push your whole leg backwards as far as you can.'

Clinical tip: The hip has to move through its full range of movement – full flexion to full extension. The limb can be heavy, so the safe positioning of the clinician is an essential part of this measurement technique.

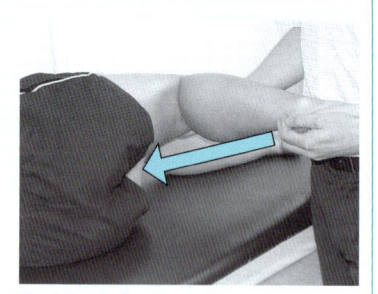

Fig 1.9 Oxford muscle grading for the hip extensors – Grade 2. The leg is moving from full hip flexion to full hip extension (backwards).

Measurement 21

Grade 3 – 'Full ROM against the effects of gravity'

Patient's position: The patient is positioned in prone lying on the plinth with their right leg over the edge of plinth so that full flexion of the hip/leg is obtained.

Clinician's position: The clinician is kneeling or standing at the side of the patient to observe the movement.

Command to patient: 'Move your leg upwards as far as you can.'

The hip has to move through its full range of movement – full flexion to full extension.

Clinical tip: You may have to commence with the hip in the neutral position, with the patient lying prone on the plinth, especially for the less able patient.

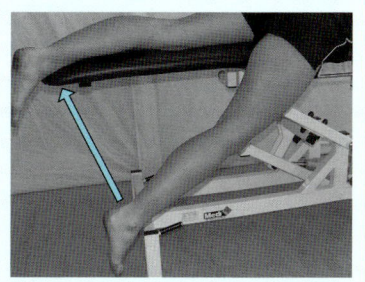

Fig 1.10 Oxford muscle grading for the hip extensors – Grade 3. The leg is moving from full hip flexion to full hip extension (towards the ceiling).

Grade 4 – 'Full ROM against minimal resistance'

Patient's position: The patient is positioned in prone lying on the plinth with the right leg over the edge of the plinth so that full flexion of the hip/leg is obtained.

Clinician's position: The clinician is standing at the foot of the plinth, applying a minimal resistance to the patient's lower leg.

Command to patient: 'Push your leg upwards as far as you can against the minimal resistance.'

The hip has to move through its full range of movement – full flexion to full extension.

Clinical tip: Use the length of lever arm principle to make sure you can apply a consistent resistance to the limb. Ask the patient to start slowly so they can appreciate the amount of resistance.

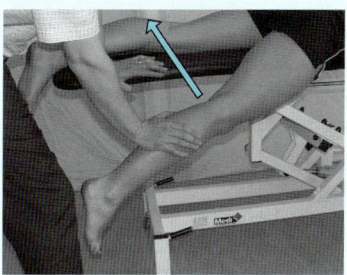

Fig 1.11 Oxford muscle grading for the hip extensors – Grades 4 and 5. The leg is moving from full hip flexion to full hip extension (towards the ceiling).

THE HIP JOINT

Grade 5 – 'Full ROM against maximal resistance'

Patient's position: The patient is positioned in prone lying on the plinth with the right leg over the edge of the plinth so that full flexion of the hip/leg is obtained (see Fig. 1.11).

Clinician's position: The clinician is standing at the foot of the plinth, applying a maximal resistance to the patient's lower leg.

Command to patient: 'Push your leg upwards as far as you can against the maximal resistance.'

The hip has to move through its full range of movement – full flexion to full extension.

Clinical tip: Use the length of lever arm principle to make sure you can apply a consistent resistance to the limb. Ask the patient to start slowly so they can appreciate the amount of resistance. Remember, the patient's hip extensors (gluteus maximus) may be stronger than your applied resistance; use a safe and mechanically advantageous position to enable you to perform this technique safely and effectively.

Flexors

Grade 0 – 'No contraction' and Grade 1 – 'Flicker of a contraction'

Patient's position: The patient is positioned in supine lying on the plinth.

Clinician's position: The clinician is standing by the patient with both hands palpating the rectus femoris muscle.

Command to patient: 'Try and tighten your thigh muscles.'/'Try and lift your leg up off the plinth.'

Clinical tip: Closely observing and feeling the muscle is essential in enabling the clinician to pick up on even the smallest flicker of a contraction.

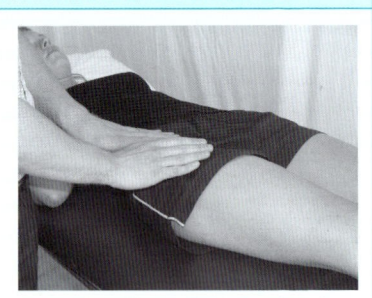

Fig 1.12 Oxford muscle grading for the hip flexors – Grades 0 and 1.

Measurement

Grade 2 – 'Full ROM with the effects of gravity eliminated'

Patient's position: The patient is positioned in side lying on the plinth. Their leg is supported in full hip extension.

Clinician's position: The clinician is standing in front of the patient, supporting the right limb with one hand under the thigh/knee and the other supporting around the foot.

Command to patient: 'Try and move your leg forwards as far as you can.'

The hip has to move through its full range of movement – full extension to full flexion.

Clinical tip: The limb can be heavy, so the safe positioning of the clinician is an essential part of this measurement technique.

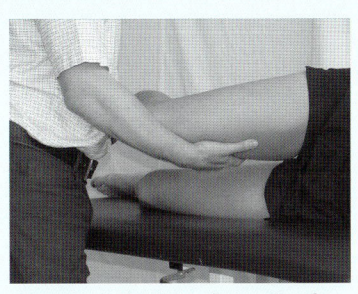

Fig 1.13 Oxford muscle grading for the hip flexors – Grade 2. The leg is moving from full hip extension to full hip flexion (forwards).

Grade 3 – 'Full ROM against the effects of gravity'

Patient's position: The patient is positioned in supine lying on the plinth, with the right leg over the edge of the plinth so that full extension of the hip/leg is obtained.

Clinician's position: The clinician is standing at the side of the patient to observe the movement.

Command to patient: 'Push your leg upwards as far as you can.'

The hip has to move through its full range of movement – full extension to full flexion.

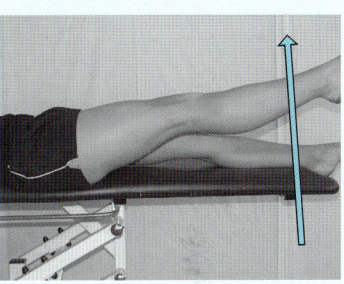

Fig 1.14 Oxford muscle grading for the hip flexors – Grade 3. The leg is moving from full hip extension to full hip flexion (towards the ceiling).

THE HIP JOINT

Grade 4 – 'Full ROM against minimal resistance'

Patient's position: The patient is positioned in supine lying on the plinth, with the right leg over the edge of the plinth so that full flexion of the hip/leg is obtained.

Clinician's position: The clinician is standing by the side of the patient, applying a minimal resistance to the patient's upper leg.

Command to patient: 'Push your leg upwards as far as you can against the minimal resistance.'

The hip has to move through its full range of movement – full extension to full flexion.

Clinical tip: Use the length of lever arm principle to make sure you can apply a consistent resistance to the limb. Ask the patient to start slowly so they can appreciate the amount of resistance.

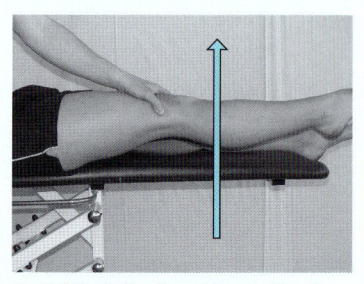

Fig 1.15 Oxford muscle grading for the hip flexors – Grades 4 and 5. The leg is moving from full hip extension to full hip flexion (towards the ceiling).

Grade 5 – 'Full ROM against maximal resistance'

Patient's position: The patient is positioned in supine lying on the plinth with the right leg over the edge of the plinth so that full flexion of the hip/leg is obtained (see Fig. 1.15).

Clinician's position: The clinician is standing by the side of the patient, applying a maximal resistance to the patient's upper leg.

Command to patient: 'Push your leg upwards as far as you can against the maximal resistance.'

The hip has to move through its full range of movement – full extension to full flexion.

Clinical tip: Use the length of lever arm principle to make sure you can apply a consistent resistance to the limb. Ask the patient to start slowly so they can appreciate the amount of resistance. Remember, the patient's hip flexors (iliopsoas and rectus femoris) may be stronger than your applied resistance. Use a safe and mechanically advantageous position to enable you to perform this technique safely and effectively.

Measurement

Abductors

Grade 0 – 'No contraction' and Grade 1 – 'Flicker of a contraction'

Patient's position: The patient is positioned in supine lying on the plinth.

Clinician's position: The clinician is standing by the patient, with both hands palpating the gluteus medius and minimus muscles.

Command to patient: 'Try and push your leg out to the side.'

Clinical tip: Closely observing and feeling the muscles is essential in enabling the clinician to pick up on even the smallest flicker of a contraction.

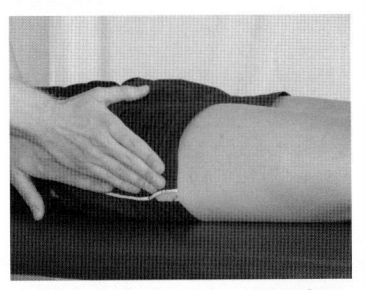

Fig 1.16 Oxford muscle grading for the hip abductors – Grades 0 and 1.

NB: Gluteus medius can be palpated between the iliac crest and the greater trochanter, whereas gluteus minimus can be palpated between the anterior superior iliac spine (ASIS) and the greater trochanter.

Grade 2 – 'Full ROM with the effects of gravity eliminated'

Patient's position: The patient is positioned in supine lying on the plinth. Their opposite leg is in abduction over the side of the plinth and the foot is resting on a stool.

Clinician's position: The clinician is standing by the patient, supporting the right limb with one hand under the thigh and the other supporting just below the knee.

Command to patient: 'Try and push your leg out to the side as far as you can.'

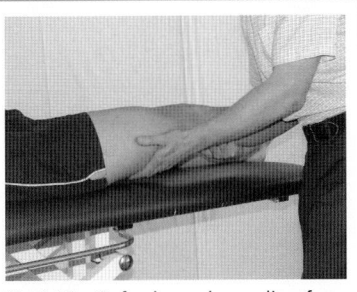

Fig 1.17 Oxford muscle grading for the hip abductors – Grade 2. The leg is moving from full hip adduction to full hip abduction (moving out sideways).

The hip has to move through its full range of movement – full adduction to full abduction.

Clinical tip: The limb can be heavy, so the safe positioning of the clinician is an essential part of this measurement technique.

THE HIP JOINT

Grade 3 – 'Full ROM against the effects of gravity'

Patient's position: The patient is positioned in side lying on the plinth or standing with the support of the plinth.

Clinician's position: The clinician is standing by the side of the patient to observe the movement.

Command to patient: If positioned in side lying – 'Push upwards with your whole leg as far as you can.'

The hip has to move through its full available range of movement – adduction to full abduction.

As the patient is positioned in side lying, the movement cannot start in full hip adduction.

If standing – 'Push your leg out to the side as far as you can.'

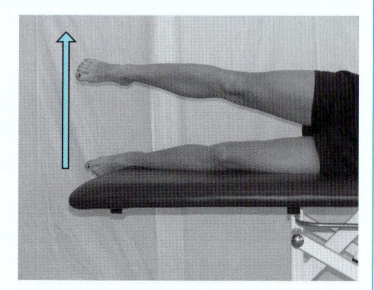

Fig 1.18 Oxford muscle grading for the hip abductors – Grade 3. The leg is moving from hip adduction to full hip abduction (towards the ceiling).

Grade 4 – 'Full ROM against minimal resistance'

Patient's position: The patient is positioned in side lying on the plinth. An alternative position is for the patient to be standing with the support of the plinth.

Clinician's position: The clinician is standing at the foot of the patient, applying a minimal resistance to the patient's lower leg.

Command to patient: 'Push your leg upwards as far as you can against the minimal resistance.'

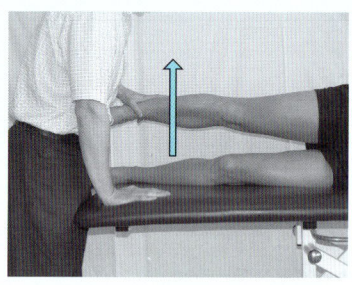

Fig 1.19 Oxford muscle grading for the hip abductors – Grades 4 and 5. The leg is moving from hip adduction to full hip abduction (towards the ceiling).

The hip has to move through its full available range of movement – adduction to full abduction.

As the patient is positioned in side lying, the movement cannot start in full hip adduction.

Clinical tip: Use the length of lever arm principle to make sure you can apply a consistent resistance to the limb. Ask the patient to start slowly so they can appreciate the amount of resistance.

Measurement 27

Grade 5 – 'Full ROM against maximal resistance'

Patient's position: The patient is positioned in side lying on the plinth or standing with the support of the plinth (see Fig. 1.19).

Clinician's position: The clinician is standing at the foot of the patient, applying a maximal resistance to the patient's lower leg.

Command to patient: 'Push your leg upwards as far as you can against the maximal resistance.'

The hip has to move through its full available range of movement – adduction to full abduction.

Clinical tip: Use the length of lever arm principle to make sure you can apply a consistent resistance to the limb. Ask the patient to start slowly so they can appreciate the amount of resistance. Remember, the patient's hip abductors (gluteus medius and minimus) may be stronger than your applied resistance. Use a safe and mechanically advantageous position to enable you to perform this technique safely and effectively.

Adductors

Grade 0 – 'No contraction' and Grade 1 – 'Flicker of a contraction'

Patient's position: The patient is positioned in supine lying on the plinth.

Clinician's position: The clinician is standing by the patient, palpating the adductor muscles (adductors magnus, longus and brevis).

Command to patient: 'Try and brace your two legs together to tighten your muscles.'

Clinical tip: Closely observing and feeling the muscle is essential in enabling the clinician to pick up on even the smallest flicker of a contraction. The adductors may be felt high up on the inside of the thigh. Adductor magnus can be palpated more easily just above the adductor tubercle of the femur on the lower, medial aspect of the femur.

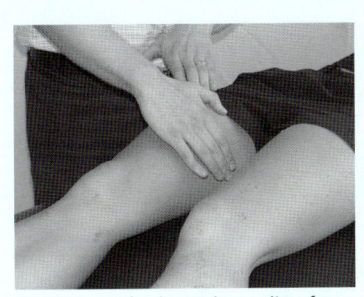

Fig 1.20 Oxford muscle grading for the hip adductors – Grades 0 and 1.

THE HIP JOINT

Grade 2 – 'Full ROM with the effects of gravity eliminated'

Patient's position: The patient is positioned in supine lying on the plinth with their right leg in abduction.

Clinician's position: The clinician is standing by the side of the patient, supporting the weight of the right limb, allowing the patient to move the hip joint into adduction.

Command to patient: 'Try and push your leg inwards as far as you can.'

The hip has to move through its full range of movement – full abduction to full adduction.

Clinical tip: The limb can be heavy, so the safe positioning of the clinician is an essential part of this measurement technique.

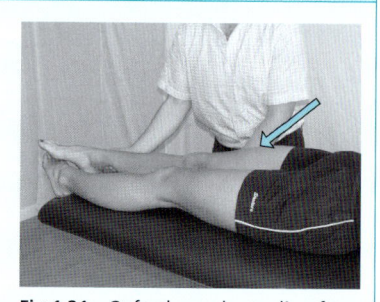

Fig 1.21 Oxford muscle grading for the hip adductors – Grade 2. The leg has moved from full hip abduction to full hip adduction (inwards).

Grade 3 – 'Full ROM against the effects of gravity'

Patient's position: The patient is positioned in right side lying on the plinth, their right hip slightly flexed to gain adduction.

Clinician's position: The clinician is standing by the side of the patient to observe the movement.

Command to patient: 'Push your leg upwards as far as you can.'

The hip has to move through its full available range of movement – abduction to full adduction.

Clinical tip: As the patient is positioned in side lying, the movement cannot start in full hip abduction.

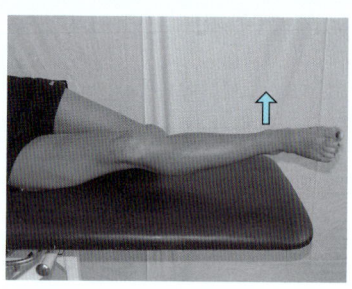

Fig 1.22 Oxford muscle grading for the hip adductors – Grade 3. The leg is moving from hip abduction to full hip adduction (towards the ceiling).

Measurement

Grade 4 – 'Full ROM against minimal resistance'

Patient's position: The patient is positioned in right side lying on the plinth, their right hip slightly flexed to gain adduction.

Clinician's position: The clinician is standing at the foot of the patient, applying a minimal resistance to the patient's lower leg.

Command to patient: 'Push your leg upwards as far as you can against the minimal resistance.'

The hip has to move through its full available range of movement – abduction to full adduction.

Clinical tip: As the patient is positioned in side lying, the movement cannot start in full hip abduction.

Clinical tip: Use the length of lever arm principle to make sure you can apply a consistent resistance to the limb. Ask the patient to start slowly so they can appreciate the amount of resistance.

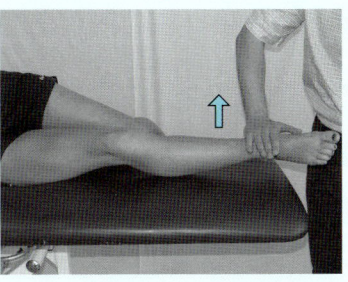

Fig 1.23 Oxford muscle grading for the hip adductors – Grades 4 and 5. The leg is moving from hip abduction to full hip adduction (towards the ceiling).

Grade 5 – 'Full ROM against maximal resistance'

Patient's position: The patient is positioned in right side lying on the plinth, their right hip slightly flexed to gain adduction (see Fig. 1.23).

Clinician's position: The clinician is standing at the foot of the patient, applying a maximal resistance to the patient's lower leg.

Command to patient: 'Push your leg upwards against the maximal resistance.'

The hip has to move through its full available range of movement – abduction to full adduction.

Clinical tip: As the patient is positioned in side lying, the movement cannot start in full hip abduction.

Clinical tip: Use the length of lever arm principle to make sure you can apply a consistent resistance to the limb. Ask the patient to start slowly so they can appreciate the amount of resistance. Remember, the patient's hip adductors (adductors magnus, longus and brevis) may be stronger than your applied resistance. Use a safe and mechanically advantageous position to enable you to perform this technique safely and effectively.

THE HIP JOINT

Lateral (external) rotators

Grade 0 – 'No contraction' and Grade 1 – 'Flicker of a contraction'

Patient's position: The patient is positioned in prone lying on the plinth.

Clinician's position: The clinician is standing by the patient with both hands palpating the gluteus maximus muscle.

Command to patient: 'Try and tighten your seat muscles.'

Clinical tip: Closely observing and feeling the muscle is essential in enabling the clinician to pick up on even the smallest flicker of a contraction. Only gluteus maximus can be palpated as the other lateral rotators are too deep.

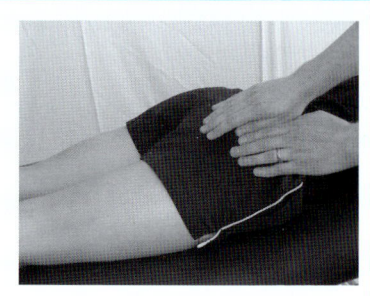

Fig 1.24 Oxford muscle grading for the hip lateral (external) rotators – Grades 0 and 1.

Grade 2 – 'Full ROM with the effects of gravity eliminated'

Patient's position: The patient is positioned in supine lying on the plinth, their leg in full medial rotation.

Clinician's position: The clinician is standing by the patient, whose leg is supported by the plinth.

Command to patient: 'Try and turn your whole leg outwards as far as you can.'

The hip has to move through its full range of movement – full medial (internal) rotation to full lateral (external) rotation.

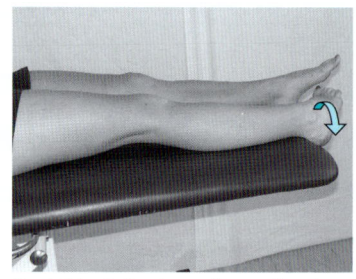

Fig 1.25 Oxford muscle grading for the hip lateral (external) rotators – Grade 2. The leg is moving from full medial rotation to full lateral rotation (leg fully turned in to leg fully turned out).

Measurement

Grade 3 – 'Full ROM against the effects of gravity'

Patient's position: The patient is positioned in sitting on the raised plinth, hip and knee in 90° of flexion. Their leg starts in full medial rotation.

Clinician's position: The clinician is standing by the side of the patient to observe the movement.

Command to patient: 'Push your leg inwards and upwards as far as you can.'

The movement commences with the patient's leg in full medial (internal) rotation and finishes in full lateral (external) rotation.

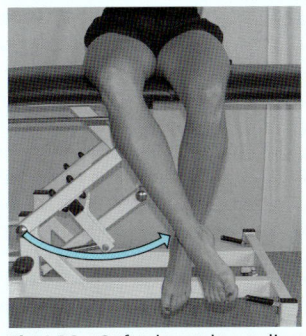

Fig 1.26 Oxford muscle grading for the hip lateral (external) rotators – Grade 3. The leg has moved from full medial rotation to full lateral rotation.

Grade 4 – 'Full ROM against minimal resistance'

Patient's position: The patient is positioned in sitting on the raised plinth, hip and knee in 90° of flexion. Their leg starts in full medial rotation.

Clinician's position: The clinician is kneeling or standing by the side of the patient, applying a minimal resistance to the patient's lower leg.

Command to patient: 'Push your leg inwards and upwards as far as you can against the minimal resistance.'

The movement commences with the patient's leg in full medial (internal) rotation and finishes in full lateral (external) rotation.

Clinical tip: Use the length of lever arm principle to make sure you can apply a consistent resistance to the limb. Ask the patient to start slowly so they can appreciate the amount of resistance.

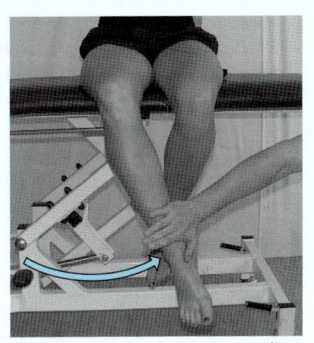

Fig 1.27 Oxford muscle grading for the hip lateral (external) rotators – Grades 4 and 5. The leg has moved from full medial rotation to full lateral rotation.

THE HIP JOINT

Grade 5 – 'Full ROM against maximal resistance'

Patient's position: The patient is positioned in sitting on the raised plinth, hip and knee in 90° of flexion. Their leg starts in full medial rotation (see Fig. 1.27).

Clinician's position: The clinician is kneeling or standing by the side of the patient, applying a maximal resistance to the patient's lower leg.

Command to patient: 'Push your leg inwards and upwards as far as you can against the maximal resistance.'

The movement commences with the patient's leg in full medial (internal) rotation and finishes in full lateral (external) rotation.

Clinical tip: Use the length of lever arm principle to make sure you can apply a consistent resistance to the limb. Ask the patient to start slowly so they can appreciate the amount of resistance. Remember, the patient's hip lateral rotators (gluteus maximus, piriformis, obturator internus, etc.) may be stronger than your applied resistance. Use a safe and mechanically advantageous position to enable you to perform this technique safely and effectively.

Medial (internal) rotators

Grade 0 – 'No contraction' and Grade 1 – 'Flicker of a contraction'

Patient's position: The patient is positioned in supine lying on the plinth.

Clinician's position: The clinician is standing by the patient with both hands palpating the gluteus medius and minimus muscles.

Command to patient: 'Try and turn your leg inwards.'

Clinical tip: Closely observing and feeling the muscles is essential in enabling the clinician to pick up on even the smallest flicker of a contraction.

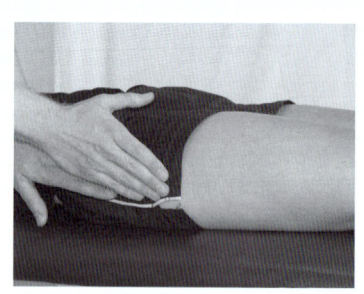

Fig 1.28 Oxford muscle grading for the hip medial (internal) rotators – Grades 0 and 1.

NB: Gluteus medius can be palpated between the iliac crest and the greater trochanter. Gluteus minimus can be palpated between the anterior superior iliac spine (ASIS) and the greater trochanter.

Measurement 33

Grade 2 – 'Full ROM with the effects of gravity eliminated'

Patient's position: The patient is positioned in supine lying on the plinth, their leg in full lateral rotation.

Clinician's position: The clinician is standing by the patient, whose leg is supported by the plinth.

Command to patient: 'Try and turn your whole leg inwards as far as you can.'

The hip has to move through its full range of movement – full lateral (external) rotation to full medial (internal) rotation.

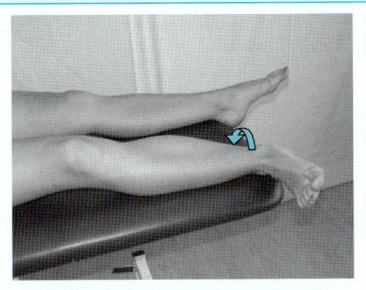

Fig 1.29 Oxford muscle grading for the hip medial (internal) rotators – Grade 2. The leg is about to move from full lateral rotation to full medial rotation (leg fully turned out to leg fully turned in).

Grade 3 – 'Full ROM against the effects of gravity'

Patient's position: The patient is positioned in sitting, on the raised plinth, their hip and knee in 90° of flexion and their leg in full lateral rotation.

Clinician's position: The clinician is standing by the side of the patient to observe the movement.

Command to patient: 'Push your leg outwards and upwards far as you can.'

The movement commences with the patient's leg in full lateral (external) rotation and finishes in full medial (internal) rotation.

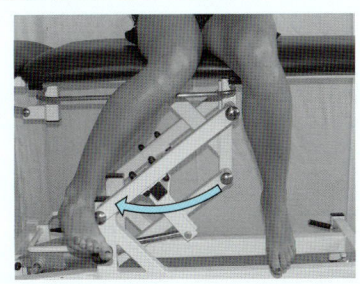

Fig 1.30 Oxford muscle grading for the hip medial (internal) rotators – Grade 3. The leg has moved from full lateral rotation to full medial rotation.

THE HIP JOINT

Grade 4 – 'Full ROM against minimal resistance'

Patient's position: The patient is positioned in sitting, on the raised plinth, hip and knee in 90° of flexion and their leg in full lateral rotation.

Clinician's position: The clinician is kneeling or standing by the side of the patient, applying a minimal resistance to the patient's lower leg.

Command to patient: 'Push your leg outwards and upwards as far as you can against the minimal resistance.'

The hip has to move through its full range of movement – full lateral (external) rotation to full medial (internal) rotation.

Clinical tip: Use the length of lever arm principle to make sure you can apply a consistent resistance to the limb. Ask the patient to start slowly so they can appreciate the amount of resistance.

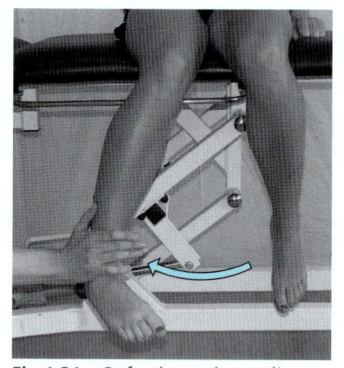

Fig 1.31 Oxford muscle grading for the hip medial (internal) rotators – Grades 4 and 5. The leg has moved from full lateral rotation to full medial rotation.

Grade 5 – 'Full ROM against maximal resistance'

Patient's position: The patient is positioned in sitting, on the raised plinth, hip and knee in 90° of flexion and their leg in full lateral rotation (see Fig. 1.31).

Clinician's position: The clinician is kneeling or standing by the side of the patient, applying a maximal resistance to the patient's lower leg.

Command to patient: 'Push your leg outwards and upwards as far as you can against the maximal resistance.'

The hip has to move through its full range of movement – full lateral (external) rotation to full medial (internal) rotation.

Clinical tip: Use the length of lever arm principle to make sure you can apply a consistent resistance to the limb. Ask the patient to start slowly so they can appreciate the amount of resistance. Remember, the patient's hip lateral rotators (gluteus medius and minimus) may be stronger than your applied resistance. Use a safe and mechanically advantageous position to enable you to perform this technique safely and effectively.

Measurement

Notes

Treatment record

LEG LENGTH

True shortening of the lower limb may occur above or below the greater trochanter, due to conditions such as coxa vara and malunion of a fracture of the shaft of the femur. Apparent shortening is a result of lateral tilting of the pelvis, secondary to conditions such as an abduction deformity of the hip joint and lumbar scoliosis. Both apparent and true discrepancies in limb length may be observed in standing, as a lateral tilting of the pelvis. Lateral tilting, due to true shortening and deformity of the hip, is eliminated if the patient sits on a hard seat, such as a gymnastic stool or a plinth. Both the lateral tilt of the pelvis and the scoliosis will still be observable if the patient has a lumbar scoliosis.

Three measurements may be performed to the medial malleolus of the tibia on each limb in order to determine the level of discrepancy (Figs 1.32, 1.33, 1.34): from the xiphisternum; from the anterior superior iliac spine (ASIS) of the innominate bone; and from the greater trochanter of the femur.

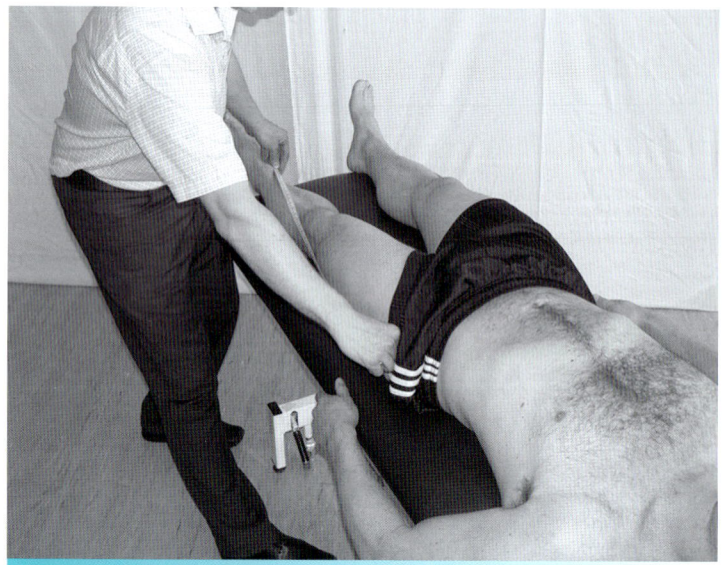

Fig 1.32 Measurement of limb length – greater trochanter of the femur to the medial malleolus of the tibia.

Measurement 37

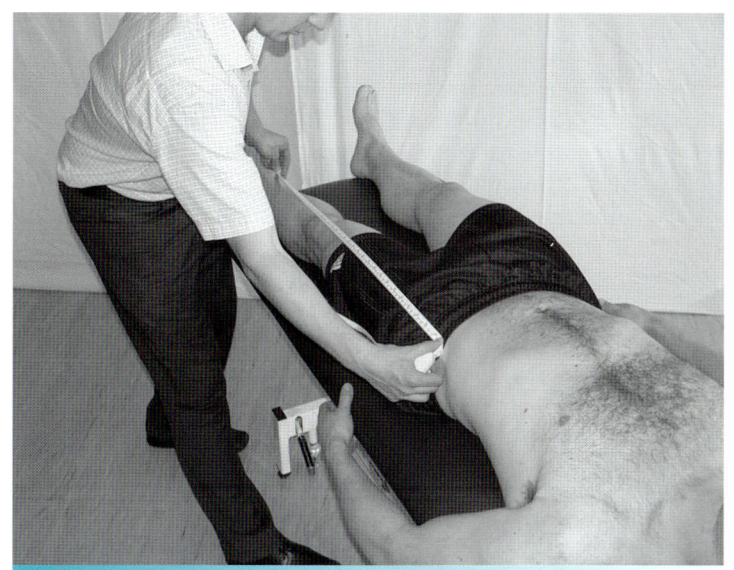

Fig 1.33 Measurement of limb length – ASIS of the innominate bone to medial malleolus of the tibia.

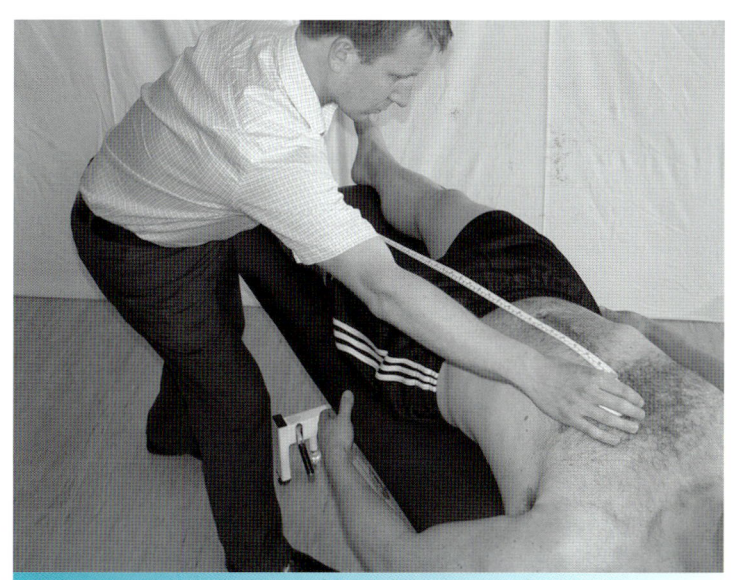

Fig 1.34 Measurement of limb length – xiphoid process to medial malleolus of the tibia.

The proximal end of the tape measure should be placed distal to the bony landmark, pushed up to it by the thumb, and held with the thumb. The distal end of the tape is held in an inferior pincer grip so that the index finger can be placed immediately distal to the medial malleolus of the tibia and the reading can be read against the thumbnail.

Patient's position: The patient is positioned in supine lying on the plinth.

Method: The clinician palpates both ASISs to determine whether or not the pelvis is set square with the lower limbs. If it is not, they must try to correct the alignment so that the limbs are in neutral and similarly disposed to the pelvis. If alignment cannot be corrected because one limb cannot be placed in neutral, the other limb must be abducted or adducted through a corresponding angle before the true length is measured.

True length of limb

This is measured from the ASIS of the innominate bone to the medial malleolus of the tibia because there is no suitable surface landmark over the centre of the acetabulum. Even if there is an abduction or adduction deformity of one hip, measurement of both limbs will be comparable as long as the other limb has been abducted or adducted to a corresponding degree.

Site of true shortening

This can be estimated by measuring from the greater trochanter of the femur to the medial malleolus of the tibia on each side. If a discrepancy is found, individual measurements should be made from the greater trochanter of the femur to the line of the knee joint and from the line of the knee joint to the medial malleolus on each limb. This will determine if there is shortening of the femur or the tibia. If there is no discrepancy in the measurements, the site of shortening is above the level of the trochanter (e.g. following fracture of the neck of the femur).

Apparent shortening

If the pelvis cannot be set square with the limbs, measurements are made from the xiphisternum to the medial malleolus of the tibia on each side with the limbs parallel. Apparent discrepancy is always due to sideways tilting of the pelvis as a result of either an abduction or an adduction deformity of the hip joint or lumbar scoliosis. Measurements from the ASIS of the innominate bone to the medial malleolus of the tibia with the limbs parallel will also be unequal.

Measurement

Notes

Treatment record

40 THE HIP JOINT

Notes

Treatment record

CHAPTER 2

The knee joint

ANATOMY 41
  Bony landmarks to be palpated 42
  Ligaments 42
  Muscles 43
    Extensors 43
    Flexors 44
    Medial (internal) rotators 45
    Lateral (external) rotators 46
MEASUREMENT 46
  Range of movement 46
    Extension 46
    Flexion 47
  Joint girth 48
    Knee 48
  Muscle bulk 49
    Limb girth: thigh 49
    Limb girth: calf 50
    Observational/reflective checklist 52
  Muscle strength: Oxford muscle grading 53
    Extensors 53
    Flexors 55

ANATOMY

1. The knee joint is one of the largest and most complex joints of the body.
2. It comprises three separate articulations: two tibiofemoral joints and the patellofemoral articulation.
3. It is a synovial, bicondylar hinge joint.
4. It has a thick capsule encapsulating all three joints which attaches to the articular margins.
5. The capsular ligaments comprise oblique popliteal ligament, the arcuate popliteal ligament and the ligamentum patellae.
6. All hinge joints have collateral ligaments. The knee joint has the tibial (medial) and fibular (lateral) collateral ligaments.
7. The intra-articular structures consist of the cruciate ligaments (anterior and posterior) and the menisci (medial and lateral).
8. The movements that take place at the knee joint are: extension and flexion. When the knee is flexed, axial rotation of the leg can be performed. These movements consist of lateral

THE KNEE JOINT

(external) rotation of the tibia on the femur and medial (internal) rotation of the tibia on the femur.

BONY LANDMARKS TO BE PALPATED

The femur – medial condyle, lateral condyle, lateral epicondyle, medial epicondyle and adductor tubercle.

The patella – anterior surface of the patella, and the apex of the patella.

The tibia – medial and lateral condyles, and the tibial tuberosity.

The fibula – the head of the fibula.

LIGAMENTS

Table 2.1

Knee ligaments

Ligament	Origin	Insertion	Limitation to movement
Anterior cruciate ligament	Anterolateral aspect of the tibia, anterior to the tibial spines on the tibial plateau	The fibres pass **u**pwards, **b**ackwards and **l**aterally to attach to the posterior part of the medial surface of the lateral femoral condyle. **AUBL** (Anterior, Upwards, Backwards, Laterally)	Limits anterior translation of the tibia on the femur
Posterior cruciate ligament	A depression in the posterior intercondylar area of the tibial plateaux	The fibres pass **u**pwards, **f**orwards and **m**edially to attach to the lateral surface of the medial condyle of the femur. **PUFM** (Posterior, Upwards, Forwards, Medially)	Limits posterior translation of the tibia on the femur
Medial collateral ligament	Medial epicondyle of the femur	Medial condyle of the tibia	Limits valgus forces of the knee
Lateral collateral ligament	Lateral epicondyle of the femur	Head of the fibula (lateral surface)	Limits varus forces of the knee
Coronary ligaments	Tibial articular margins	Meniscus	Attachment of the menisci to the tibia

MUSCLES
Extensors

Table 2.2

The extensors of the knee

Muscle	Origin	Insertion	Nerve supply	Action(s)
Rectus femoris	Straight head – anterior inferior iliac spine Reflected head – roughened area above the acetabulum of the innominate (hip) bone	Upper border of the patella, and via the ligamentum patellae to the tibial tuberosity	Femoral nerve L2, 3, 4	Flexion of the hip and extension of the knee
Vastus lateralis	Upper lateral part of the intertrochanteric line, the lower border of the greater trochanter, lateral side of the gluteal tuberosity and the upper half of the lateral lip of the linea aspera of the femur	Base and lateral border of the patella, blending with rectus femoris	Femoral nerve L2, 3, 4	Extension of the knee and acts as a stabilizer
Vastus medialis	Lower medial end of the intertrochanteric line, medial aspect of the end of the shaft on the spiral line, the medial lip of the linea aspera of the femur	Upper two-thirds of the medial supracondylar line, intermuscular septum and the tendon of adductor magnus	Femoral nerve L2, 3, 4	Extension of the knee and acts as a stabilizer
Vastus intermedius	Upper two-thirds of the anterior and lateral surface of the femur	Base of the patella, and blends with the deep aspect of the tendon of rectus femoris	Femoral nerve L2, 3, 4	Extension of the knee and acts as a stabilizer
Tensor fascia lata	Anterior one-third of the outer lip of the iliac crest of the innominate (hip) bone	Blends into the iliotibial tract, which in turn inserts into the lateral aspect of the patella tendon/retinaculum and thus the lateral aspect of the tibia	Superior gluteal nerve L4, 5	Flexion, abduction and medial rotation of the hip Extension of the knee

THE KNEE JOINT

Flexors

Table 2.3

The flexors of the knee				
Muscle	Origin	Insertion	Nerve supply	Action(s)
Biceps femoris	Ischial tuberosity of the innominate (hip) bone	Head of fibula	Sciatic nerve L5, S1, 2	Extension of the hip and flexion of the knee joint
Semimembranosus	Ischial tuberosity of the innominate (hip) bone	Posteromedial surface of medial condyle of tibia	Sciatic nerve L5, S1, 2	Extension of the hip and flexion of the knee joint
Semitendinosus	Ischial tuberosity of the innominate (hip) bone	Medial surface of medial condyle of tibia	Sciatic nerve L5, S1, 2	Extension of the hip and flexion of the knee joint
Gastrocnemius	Medial and lateral condyles of the femur	Via the Achilles tendon into the posterior surface of the calcaneus	Tibial nerve S1, 2	Plantar-flexion of the ankle joint. Flexion of the knee joint
Sartorius	Anterior superior iliac spine (ASIS) of the innominate bone	Medial side of the body of the tibia	Femoral nerve L2, 3	Flexion of the hip and knee, lateral rotation and abduction of the thigh, and medial rotation of the tibia on the femur
Gracilis	Front of the body of the pubis, inferior pubic and ischial rami of the innominate bone	Medial surface of the body of the tibia	Obturator nerve L2, 3	Adduction of the thigh and flexion of the knee joint

Anatomy

Medial (internal) rotators

Table 2.4

The medial (internal) rotators of the knee					
Muscle	Origin	Insertion	Nerve supply	Action(s)
Semimembranosus	Ischial tuberosity of the innominate (hip) bone	Posteromedial surface of medial condyle of tibia	Sciatic nerve L5, S1, 2	Extension of the hip and flexion of the knee joint
Semitendinosus	Ischial tuberosity of the innominate (hip) bone	Medial surface of medial condyle of tibia	Sciatic nerve L5, S1, 2	Extension of the hip and flexion of the knee joint
Sartorius	Anterior superior iliac spine (ASIS) of the innominate bone	Medial side of the body of the tibia	Femoral nerve L2, 3	Flexion of hip and knee, lateral rotation and abduction of the thigh, and medial rotation of the tibia on the femur
Gracilis	Front of the body of the pubis, inferior pubic and ischial rami of the innominate bone	Medial surface of the body of the tibia	Obturator nerve L2, 3	Adduction of the thigh and flexion of the knee joint
Popliteus	Anterior aspect of the outer surface of the lateral condyle of the femur	Posterior surface of the tibia above the soleal line	Tibial nerve L5	Lateral rotation of the femur on the tibia, unlocking the knee from the close-packed position

THE KNEE JOINT

Lateral (external) rotators

Table 2.5

The lateral (external) rotators of the knee

Muscle	Origin	Insertion	Nerve supply	Action(s)
Biceps femoris	Ischial tuberosity of the innominate (hip) bone	Head of fibula	Sciatic nerve L5, S1, 2	Extension of the hip and flexion and lateral rotation of the knee

MEASUREMENT

RANGE OF MOVEMENT
Extension

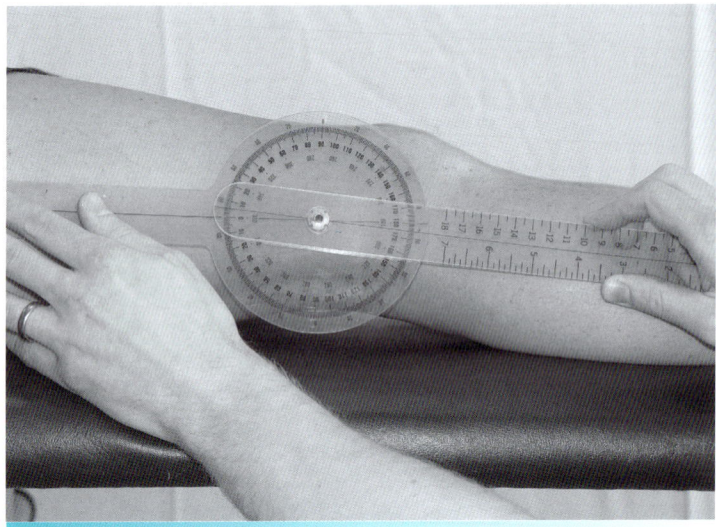

Fig 2.1 Goniometric measurement of knee extension.

Starting position: The patient is positioned in half lying/supine lying on the plinth, their hip in neutral and their knee in extension.
Goniometer axis: The axis of the goniometer is placed over the lateral epicondyle of the femur.
Stationary arm: This is parallel to the longitudinal axis of the femur, pointing towards the greater trochanter of the femur.

Moveable arm: This is parallel to the longitudinal axis of the fibula, pointing towards the lateral malleolus of the fibula.
Command to patient: 'Straighten your leg as much as possible.'
End position: The knee is extended to its limit of motion.

Flexion

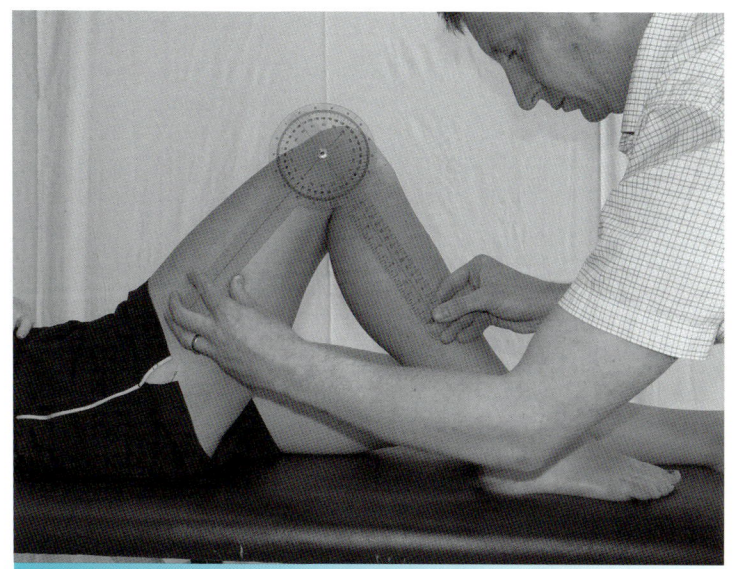

Fig 2.2 Goniometric measurement of knee flexion.

Starting position: The patient is positioned in half lying/supine lying on the plinth. Their hip is in neutral and their knee is in extension.
Goniometer axis: The axis of the goniometer is placed over the lateral epicondyle of the femur.
Stationary arm: This is parallel to the longitudinal axis of the femur, pointing towards the greater trochanter of the femur.
Moveable arm: This is parallel to the longitudinal axis of the fibula, pointing towards the lateral malleolus of the fibula.
Command to patient: 'Bend your knee up towards you so that your heel moves towards your buttock as much as possible.'
End position: The hip and knee are flexed to the limit of motion. The heel is moved towards the buttock to the limit of knee flexion.

> NB: It may be necessary to reposition the stationary and moveable arms of the goniometer prior to taking the reading, as they may have moved when the patient flexed their knee.

THE KNEE JOINT

JOINT GIRTH
Knee

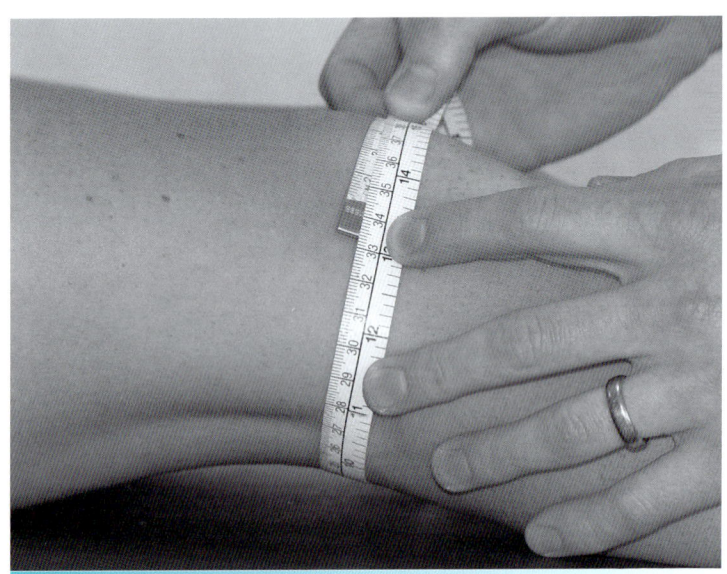

Fig 2.3 Measurement of the girth of the knee joint.

Patient's position: The patient is positioned in half lying or supine lying on the plinth.

Method: The knee joint girth can be measured by taking a circumferential measurement with a tape measure around the knee joint line. (The knee joint line can be identified by following either side of the patella tendon up from the tibial tuberosity with the knee in 45–90° of flexion. The relatively wide anterior aspect of the joint line can be palpated and followed around to the lateral and medial joint margins.)

Repeat three times and produce an average reading.

Repeat the procedure on the other limb to compare the two measurements.

Points to note:
  The state of the tape measure – is it stretched?
  The muscles must be relaxed.
  Keep the tape measure straight (not twisted).
  Measure consistently – at the top/bottom of the tape, and
    either in centimetres or in inches.

MUSCLE BULK
Limb girth: thigh

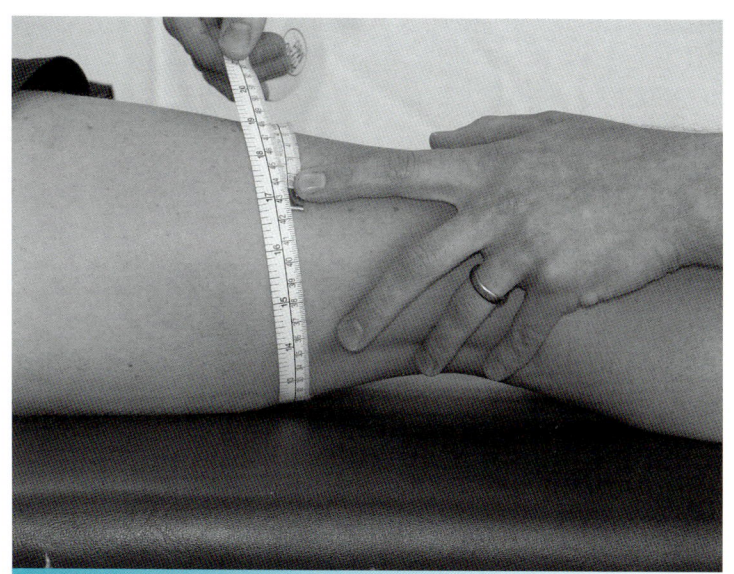

Fig 2.4 Measurement of the girth of the thigh.

Patient's position: The patient is positioned in long sitting/half lying on the plinth, well supported. The knees are in passive extension so that the thigh and calf muscles are relaxed.

Method: Three points are marked – 15 cm (6 inches), 20 cm (8 inches) and 25 cm (10 inches) above the distal end of the tibial tuberosity. The limb is encircled with a tape measure at each marked point. The circumferential measurements are then recorded.

Repeat three times and produce an average reading, then repeat the procedure on the other limb to compare the two measurements.

Points to note:
  The state of the tape measure – is it stretched?
  The muscles must be relaxed.
  Keep the tape measure straight (not twisted).
  Measure consistently – at the top/bottom of the tape, and either in centimetres or in inches.

THE KNEE JOINT

Limb girth: calf

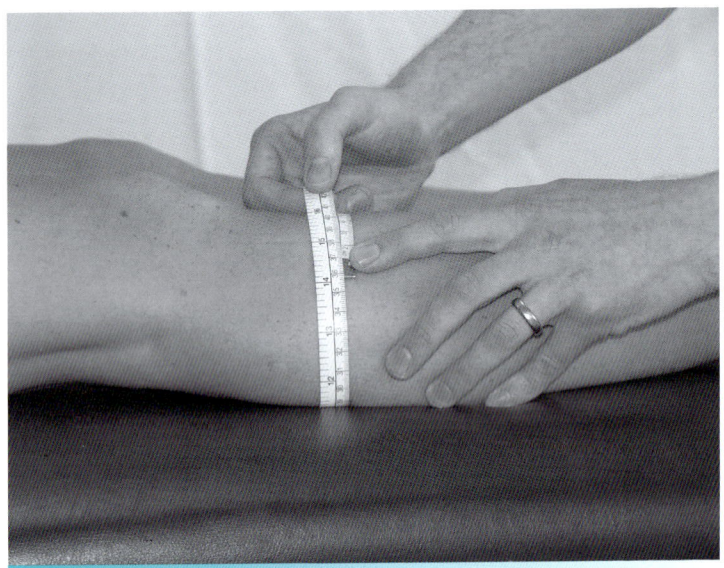

Fig 2.5 Measurement of the girth of the calf.

Patient's position: The patient is positioned in long sitting/half lying on the plinth, well supported. The knees are in passive extension so that the calf and thigh muscles are relaxed.
Method: Mark two or three points – 5 cm (2 inches), 10 cm (4 inches), and 15 cm (6 inches) below the distal end of the tibial tuberosity. If the patient is small in stature, the measurement at 15 cm (6 inches) may not be necessary. The limb is encircled with a tape measure at each marked point. The circumferential measurements are then recorded.

Repeat the procedure three times and produce an average reading.

Repeat the procedure on the other limb to compare the results.

Points to note:
  The state of the tape measure – is it stretched?
  The muscles must be relaxed.
  Keep the tape measure straight (not twisted).
  Measure consistently – at the top/bottom of the tape, and
    either in centimetres or in inches.

Measurement 51

Notes

Treatment record

THE KNEE JOINT

Observational/reflective checklist

Observational/reflective checklist			
Observation		Y/N	Comments
Introduction and preparation for the skill	Was the treatment area properly prepared for the patient, e.g. pillow, blanket, safe environment, etc.?		
	Did the therapist introduce him/herself?		
	Was the patient comfortable?		
	Was the patient adequately exposed/draped?		
	Was an explanation of the procedure given?		
	Was the explanation clear and succinct?		
	Was consent obtained?		
Performing the skill	Was the plinth set at the correct height?		
	Was the therapist's posture compromised?		
	Did the therapist identify the joint and other relevant bony landmarks?		
	Was the tape measure correctly aligned?		
	Was the reading of the limb girth accurate?		
	Did the therapist compare both sides of the body?		
Safe and effective performance of the technique	Was the procedure carried out with due care and attention?		
How would you rate the proficiency in the overall performance of the skill?	Excellent		
	Very good		
	Good		
	Satisfactory		
	Borderline		
	Fail		

Measurement

MUSCLE STRENGTH: OXFORD MUSCLE GRADING

Extensors

Grade 0 – 'No contraction' and Grade 1 – 'Flicker of a contraction'

Patient's position: The patient is positioned in long sitting on the plinth.

Clinician's position: The clinician is standing by the patient, with both hands palpating the quadriceps muscles (vastus medialis and vastus lateralis) for a contraction.

Command to patient: 'Try and tighten your thigh muscles.'

Clinical tip: Closely observing and feeling the muscle is essential in enabling the clinician to pick up on even the smallest flicker of a contraction.

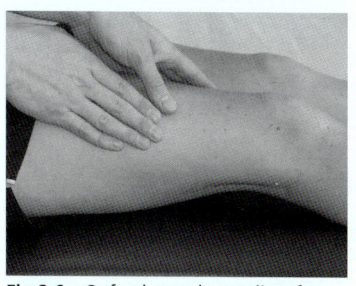

Fig 2.6 Oxford muscle grading for the knee extensors – Grades 0 and 1.

Grade 2 – 'Full ROM with the effects of gravity eliminated'

Patient's position: The patient is positioned in side lying on the plinth. Their leg is supported in full knee flexion.

Clinician's position: The clinician is standing by the patient, supporting the right limb, with one hand under the thigh and the other supporting just below the knee.

Command to patient: 'Try and straighten your leg as far as you can.'

The knee has to move through its full range of movement – full flexion to full extension.

Clinical tip: The limb can be heavy, so the safe positioning of the clinician is an essential part of this measurement technique.

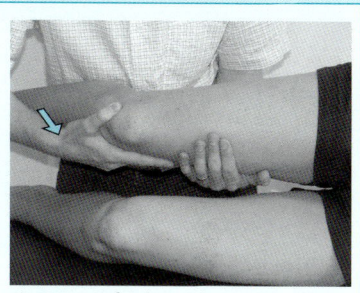

Fig 2.7 Oxford muscle grading for the knee extensors – Grade 2. The knee is moving from full flexion to full extension (the leg is straightening).

THE KNEE JOINT

Grade 3 – 'Full ROM against the effects of gravity'

Patient's position: The patient is positioned in sitting over the edge of the plinth so that full flexion of the knee is obtained.

Clinician's position: The clinician is kneeling by the patient to observe the movement.

Command to patient: 'Straighten your leg as far as you can.'

The knee has to move through its full range of movement – full flexion to full extension.

Clinical tip: This position does compromise the movement from full flexion, because of the effects of gravity; however, practically it is one of the most suitable positions and allows easy progress to testing for Grades 4 and 5.

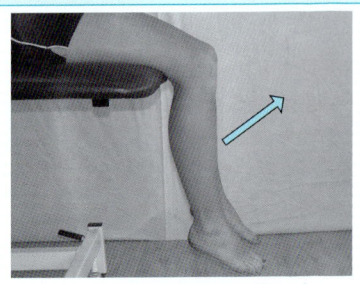

Fig 2.8 Oxford muscle grading for the knee extensors – Grade 3. The knee is moving from full flexion to full extension (the leg is straightening).

Grade 4 – 'Full ROM against minimal resistance'

Patient's position: The patient is positioned in sitting over the edge of the plinth so that full flexion of the knee is obtained.

Clinician's position: The clinician is kneeling in front of the patient, applying a minimal resistance to the patient's lower leg.

Command to patient: 'Straighten your leg as far as you can against the minimal resistance.'

The knee has to move through its full range of movement – full flexion to full extension.

Clinical tip: Use the length of lever arm principle to make sure you can apply a consistent resistance to the limb. Ask the patient to start slowly so they can appreciate the amount of resistance.

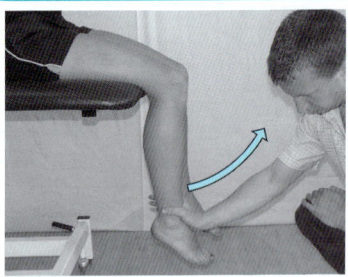

Fig 2.9 Oxford muscle grading for the knee extensors – Grades 4 and 5. The knee is moving from full flexion to full extension (the leg is straightening).

Measurement 55

Grade 5 – 'Full ROM against maximal resistance'

Patient's position: The patient is positioned in sitting over the edge of the plinth so that full flexion of the knee is obtained (see Fig. 2.9).

Clinician's position: The clinician is kneeling in front of the patient, applying a maximal resistance to the patient's lower leg.

Command to patient: 'Straighten your leg as far as you can against the maximal resistance.'

The knee has to move through its full range of movement – full flexion to full extension.

Clinical tip: Use the length of lever arm principle to make sure you can apply a consistent resistance to the limb. Ask the patient to start slowly so they can appreciate the amount of resistance. Remember, the patient's quadriceps may be stronger than your applied resistance. Use a safe and mechanically advantageous position to enable you to perform this technique safely and effectively.

Flexors

Grade 0 – 'No contraction' and Grade 1 – 'Flicker of a contraction'

Patient's position: The patient is positioned in prone lying on the plinth.

Clinician's position: The clinician is standing by the side of the patient with both hands palpating the hamstring muscles (semimembranosus, semitendinosus, biceps femoris) for a contraction.

Command to patient: 'Try and tighten your posterior thigh muscles.'

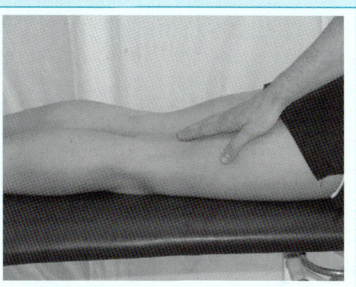

Fig 2.10 Oxford muscle grading for the knee flexors – Grades 0 and 1.

Clinical tip: Closely observing and feeling the muscles is essential in enabling the clinician to pick up on even the smallest flicker of a contraction.

THE KNEE JOINT

Grade 2 – 'Full ROM with the effects of gravity eliminated'

Patient's position: The patient is positioned in side lying on the plinth. Their leg is supported in full knee extension.

Clinician's position: The clinician is standing by the patient, supporting the right limb with one hand under the thigh/ knee and the other supporting just above the ankle.

Command to patient: 'Try and bend your leg backwards as far as you can.'

The knee has to move through its full range of movement – full extension to full flexion.

Clinical tip: The limb can be heavy, so the safe positioning of the clinician is an essential part of this measurement technique.

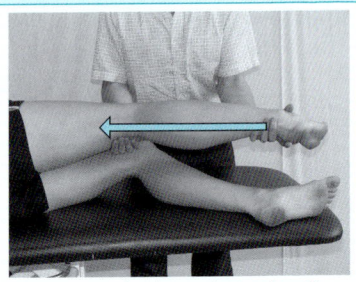

Fig 2.11 Oxford muscle grading for the knee flexors – Grade 2. The knee is moving from full extension to full flexion (the heel is moving backwards towards the buttock).

Grade 3 – 'Full ROM against the effects of gravity'

Patient's position: The patient is positioned in standing, using the plinth for support.

Clinician's position: The clinician is standing by the patient to observe the movement.

Command to patient: 'Bend your leg up as far as you can.'

The knee has to move through its full range of movement – full extension to full flexion.

Clinical tip: The more unstable patient may have to be positioned in prone lying on the plinth. In this position full knee flexion will be completed with the effects of gravity assisting the movement, i.e. after 90° of knee flexion has been achieved.

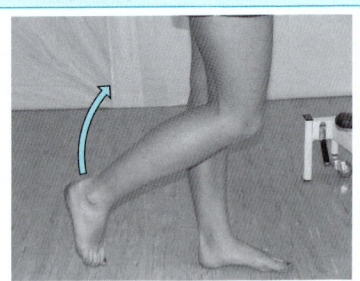

Fig 2.12 Oxford muscle grading for the knee flexors – Grade 3. The knee is moving from full extension to full flexion (the heel is moving up towards the buttock).

Measurement

Grade 4 – 'Full ROM against minimal resistance'

Patient's position: The patient is positioned in prone lying on the plinth with their right foot over the end of the plinth so that full extension of the knee is obtained.

Clinician's position: The clinician is standing to the side of the patient, applying a minimal resistance to the patient's lower leg.

Command to patient: 'Bend your leg up as far as you can against the minimal resistance.'

The knee has to move through its full range of movement – full extension to full flexion.

Clinical tip: Use the length of lever arm principle to make sure you can apply a consistent resistance to the limb. Ask the patient to start slowly so they can appreciate the amount of resistance.

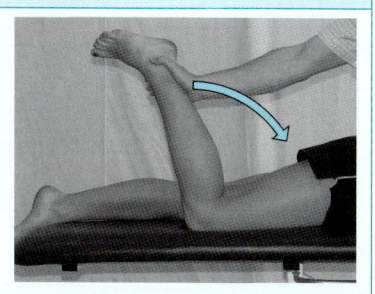

Fig 2.13 Oxford muscle grading for the knee flexors – Grades 4 and 5. The knee is moving from full extension to full flexion (the heel is moving towards the buttock).

Grade 5 – 'Full ROM against maximal resistance'

Patient's position: The patient is positioned in prone lying with their right foot over the end of the plinth so that full extension of the knee is obtained (see Fig. 2.13).

Clinician's position: The clinician is standing to the side of the patient, applying a maximal resistance to the patient's lower leg.

Command to patient: 'Bend your leg up as far as you can against the maximal resistance.'

The knee has to move through its full range of movement – full extension to full flexion.

Clinical tip: Use the length of lever arm principle to make sure you can apply a consistent resistance to the limb. Ask the patient to start slowly so they can appreciate the amount of resistance. Remember, the patient's hamstrings may be stronger than your applied resistance. Use a safe and mechanically advantageous position to enable you to perform this technique safely and effectively.

58   THE KNEE JOINT

Notes

Treatment record

CHAPTER 3

The ankle joint

ANATOMY 59
  Bony landmarks to be palpated 59
  Ligaments 60
  Muscles 61
    Plantarflexors 61
    Dorsiflexors 62
    Invertors 63
    Evertors 64
MEASUREMENT 65
  Range of movement 65
    Dorsiflexion 65
    Plantarflexion 66

    Inversion 67
    Eversion 69
    Observational/reflective checklist 71
  Joint girth 72
  Limb girth 75
    Calf 75
  Muscle strength: Oxford muscle grading 77
    Plantarflexors 77
    Dorsiflexors 79
    Evertors 82
    Invertors 84

ANATOMY

1. The ankle joint is a synovial hinge joint.
2. It is an articulation between the distal end of the tibia and fibula with the body of the talus.
3. A fibrous capsule completely surrounds the joint, attaching to the articular margins.
4. It is supported by strong lateral and medial ligaments.
5. The ankle is most stable in dorsiflexion, which is the joint's closed packed position.
6. The anterior talofibular ligament appears to be the ligament most prone to injury.
7. The movements that take place at the ankle joint are plantarflexion (flexion) and dorsiflexion (extension).

BONY LANDMARKS TO BE PALPATED

The tibia – anterior border, medial surface, and the medial malleolus.

THE ANKLE JOINT

The fibula – lateral malleolus.

The foot – the head of the talus, the sustentaculum tali of the calcaneus, the tuberosity of the navicular and the base of the 5th metatarsal.

LIGAMENTS

Table 3.1

Ankle ligaments			
Ligament	Origin	Insertion	Limitation to movement
Medial (deltoid) ligament (deep parts)			
Anterior tibiotalar band	Tip of the medial malleolus	Medial part of neck of talus	Resists the forward displacement of the foot
Posterior tibiotalar band	Tip of the medial malleolus	Medial neck of talus and medial tubercle	Resists the backward displacement of the foot
Medial (deltoid) ligament (superficial parts)			
Tibionavicular band	Tip of the medial malleolus	Tuberosity on the navicular	Resists eversion forces
Tibiocalcaneal band	Tip of the medial malleolus	Sustentaculum tali of the calcaneus bone	Resists the backward displacement of the foot
Lateral ligament			
Anterior talofibular ligament	Tip of lateral malleolus	Neck of the talus	Resists the forward displacement of the foot and inversion
Posterior talofibular ligament	Tip of lateral malleolus	Lateral tubercle of the posterior process of the talus	Resists inversion forces – and resists the backwards displacement of the foot
Calcaneofibular ligament	Tip of lateral malleolus	Peroneal tubercle on the lateral surface of the calcaneus	Resists the backwards displacement of the foot
Anterior ligament	Anterior margin of lower end of tibia	Anterior part of neck of talus	Resists the forward displacement of the foot
Posterior ligament	Posterior aspects of tibia and fibula	Medial tubercle of posterior surface of talus	Resists the backward displacement of the foot

MUSCLES
Plantarflexors

Table 3.2

Muscle	Origin	Insertion	Nerve supply	Action(s)
Gastrocnemius	Medial and lateral condyles of the femur	Via the Achilles tendon into the posterior surface of the calcaneus	Tibial nerve S1, 2	Plantarflexion of the ankle. Flexion of the knee joint
Soleus	Soleal line on posterior surface of tibia, posterior surface of upper third of fibula and fibrous arch between the two	Via the Achilles tendon into the posterior surface of the calcaneus	Tibial nerve S1, 2	Plantarflexion of the ankle, postural muscle. The soleal pump aids venous return
Plantaris	Lateral supracondylar ridge and popliteal surface of the femur	Via the Achilles tendon into the posterior surface of the calcaneus	Tibial nerve S1, 2	Weak plantarflexion of the ankle and weak flexion of the knee
Tibialis posterior	Upper half of lateral aspect of posterior surface of tibia, interosseous membrane and posterior surface of the fibula	Tubercle on medial aspect of navicular, medial cuneiform + tendinous slips to most of the tarsal bones	Tibial nerve L4, 5	Inversion of the foot and plantarflexion of the ankle
Flexor digitorum longus	Medial part of the posterior surface of the tibia	Distal phalanx of lateral four toes	Tibial nerve L5, S1, 2	Flexion of the lateral four toes. Plantarflexion of the ankle
Flexor hallucis longus	Lower two-thirds of the posterior surface of the fibula	Base of distal phalanx of the great toe	Tibial nerve S1, 2	Flexion of all the joints of the great toe

Dorsiflexors

Table 3.3

The dorsiflexors of the ankle				
Muscle	Origin	Insertion	Nerve supply	Action(s)
Tibialis anterior	Upper two-thirds of the lateral surface of tibia and the interosseous membrane	Medial side of medial cuneiform and base of the first metatarsal	Deep peroneal nerve L4, 5	Dorsiflexion of the ankle and inversion of the foot
Extensor digitorum longus	Upper two-thirds of anterior surface of fibula, interosseous membrane, and lateral condyle of the tibia	The base of the middle and distal phalanx of the lateral four toes	Deep peroneal nerve L5, S1	Extension of the lateral four toes and dorsiflexion of the ankle
Extensor hallucis longus	Middle half of the anterior surface of the fibula and the interosseous membrane	The base of the distal phalanx of the great toe	Deep peroneal nerve L5, S1	Extension of the great toe and dorsiflexion of the ankle
Peroneus tertius	Lower quarter of the fibula and the intermuscular septum	The base of the 5th metatarsal	Deep peroneal nerve L5, S1	Eversion and dorsiflexion of the ankle

Invertors

Table 3.4

The invertors of the ankle				
Muscle	Origin	Insertion	Nerve supply	Action(s)
Tibialis posterior	Upper half of lateral aspect of posterior surface of tibia, interosseous membrane and posterior surface of the fibula	Tubercle on medial aspect of navicular, medial cuneiform + tendinous slips to most of the tarsal bones	Tibial nerve L4, 5	Inversion of the foot and plantarflexion of the ankle
Tibialis anterior	Upper two-thirds of the lateral surface of tibia and the interosseous membrane	Medial side of medial cuneiform and base of the first metatarsal	Deep peroneal nerve L4, 5	Dorsiflexion of the ankle and inversion of the foot

Evertors

Table 3.5

The evertors of the ankle

Muscle	Origin	Insertion	Nerve supply	Action(s)
Peroneus longus	Upper two-thirds of the lateral surface of the fibula	Lateral surfaces of medial cuneiform and base of the first metatarsal	Superficial peroneal nerve L5, S1	Eversion of the foot, and plantarflexion of the ankle
Peroneus brevis	Lower two-thirds of lateral surface of the fibula	Base of the 5th metatarsal	Superficial peroneal nerve L5, S1	Eversion of the foot, and plantarflexion of the ankle
Peroneus tertius	Lower quarter of the fibula and the intermuscular septum	Base of the 5th metatarsal	Deep peroneal nerve L5, S1	Eversion of the foot, and dorsiflexion of the ankle

MEASUREMENT

RANGE OF MOVEMENT

Dorsiflexion

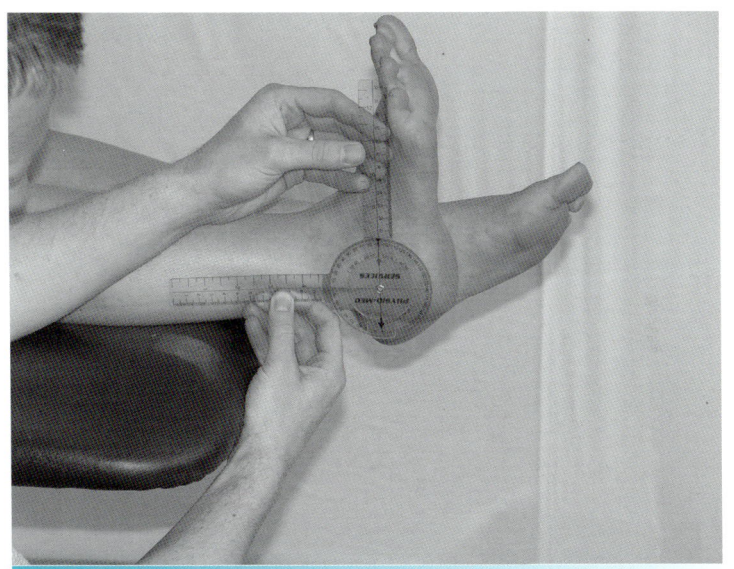

Fig 3.1 Goniometric measurement of ankle dorsiflexion.

Starting position: The patient is positioned in supine lying on the plinth, their knee is slightly flexed and their foot is in neutral – 0°.
Goniometer axis: The axis of the goniometer is placed 1.5 cm below the lateral malleolus of the fibula.
Stationary arm: This is parallel to the longitudinal axis of the fibula, in line with the head of the fibula.
Moveable arm: This is parallel to the longitudinal axis of the 5th metatarsal.
Command to patient: 'Bend your foot up as far as you can' (dorsiflexion).
End position: The ankle is dorsiflexed to the limit of motion.

NB: It may be necessary to reposition the stationary and moveable arms of the goniometer prior to taking the reading, as they may have moved when the patient dorsiflexed their ankle.

Plantarflexion

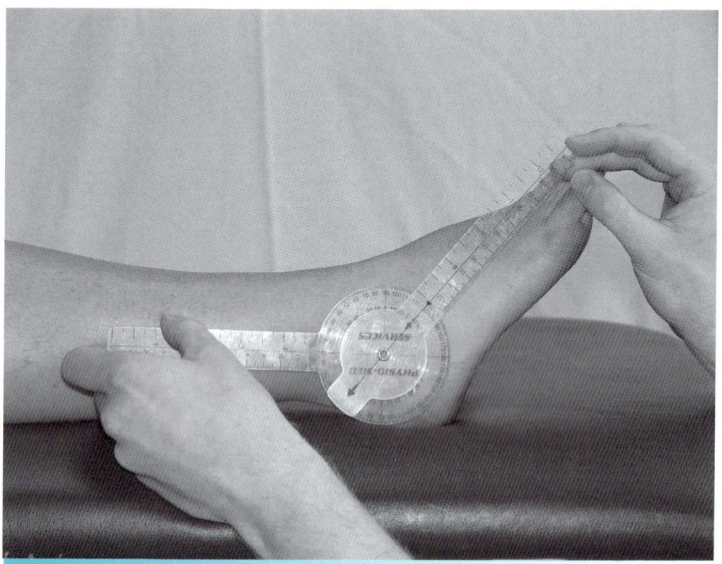

Fig 3.2 Goniometric measurement of ankle plantarflexion.

Starting position: The patient is positioned in supine lying on the plinth, their knee is slightly flexed and their foot is in neutral – 0°.
Goniometer axis: The axis of the goniometer is placed 1.5 cm below the lateral malleolus of the fibula.
Stationary arm: This is parallel to the longitudinal axis of the fibula, in line with the head of the fibula.
Moveable arm: This is parallel to the longitudinal axis of the 5th metatarsal.
Command to patient: 'Push your foot down as far as you can' (plantarflexion).
End position: The ankle is plantarflexed to the limit of motion.

Inversion

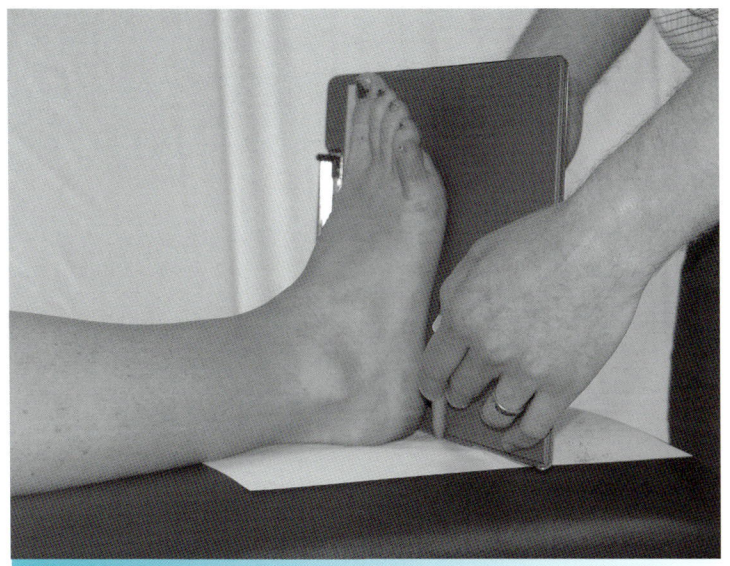

Fig 3.3 Measurement of the foot in neutral.

Starting position: The patient is positioned in supine lying on the plinth; a roll is placed under the knee. The ankle is in neutral – 0°.

A piece of paper is placed under the foot, a book is placed against the sole of the foot, and a line is drawn parallel to the book.

Command to patient: 'Turn your foot in as far as you can' (inversion).
End position: The foot has moved into inversion.

The book is placed against the full sole of the foot and a line is drawn parallel to the book. This line should bisect the original line, making an angle. This angle relates to the degree of inversion at the foot.

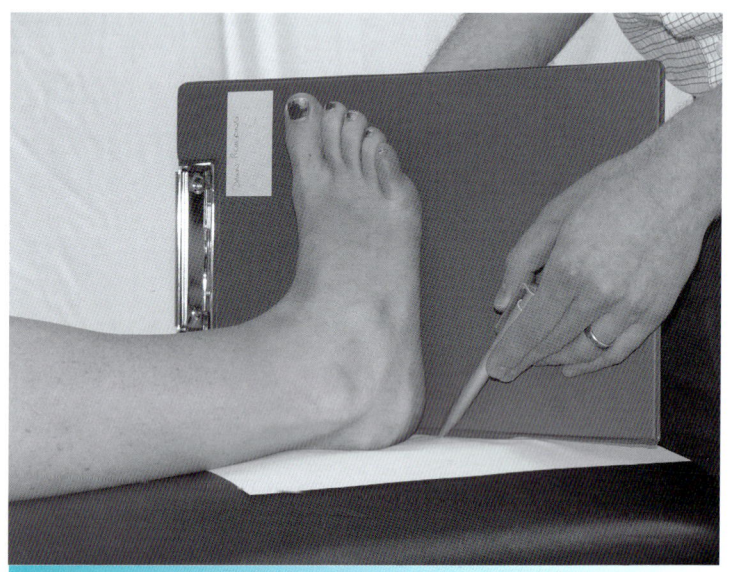

Fig 3.4 Measurement of foot inversion.

Eversion

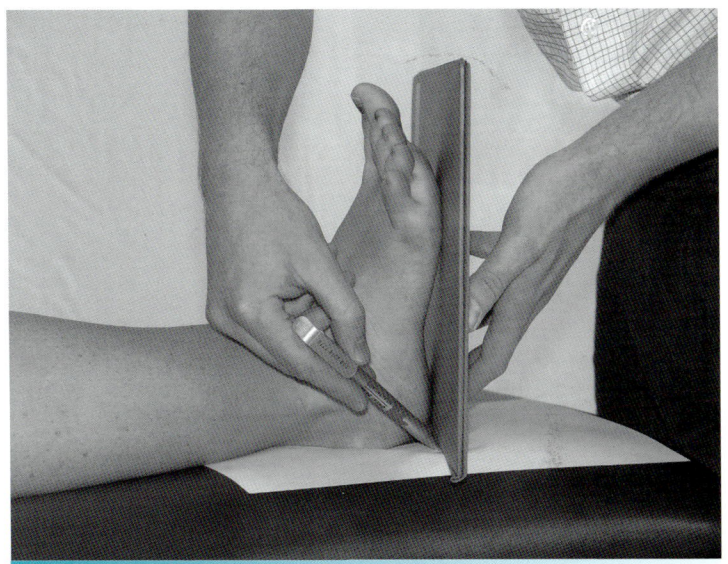

Fig 3.5 Measurement of foot eversion.

Starting position: The patient is positioned in supine lying on the plinth; a roll is placed under the knee. The ankle is in neutral – 0°.

A piece of paper is placed under the foot, a book is placed against the sole of the foot, and a line is drawn parallel to the book.

Command to patient: 'Turn your foot out as far as you can' (eversion).

End position: The foot has moved into eversion.

The book is placed against the full sole of the foot and a line is drawn parallel to the book. This line should bisect the original line, making an angle. This angle relates to the degree of eversion at the foot.

THE ANKLE JOINT

Notes

Treatment record

Observational/reflective checklist

Observational/reflective checklist			
Observation		Y/N	Comments
Introduction and preparation for the skill	Was the treatment area properly prepared for the patient, e.g. pillow, blanket, safe environment, etc.?		
	Did the therapist introduce him/herself?		
	Was the patient comfortable?		
	Was the patient adequately exposed/draped?		
	Was an explanation of the procedure given?		
	Was the explanation clear and succinct?		
	Was consent obtained?		
Performing the skill	Was the plinth set at the correct height?		
	Was the therapist's posture compromised?		
	Did the therapist identify the joint and other relevant bony landmarks?		
	Was the goniometer correctly aligned?		
	Was the reading of the joint range of movement accurate?		
	Did the therapist compare both sides of the body?		
Safe and effective performance of the technique	Was the procedure carried out with due care and attention?		
How would you rate the proficiency in the overall performance of the skill?	Excellent		
	Very good		
	Good		
	Satisfactory		
	Borderline		
	Fail		

THE ANKLE JOINT

JOINT GIRTH

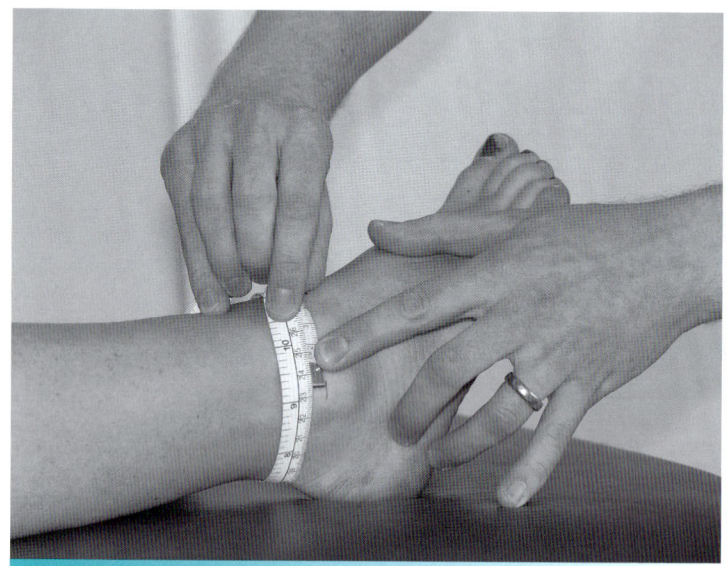

Fig 3.6 Measurement of the girth of the ankle joint.

Patient's position: The patient is positioned in half lying or supine lying on the plinth.
Method: The ankle joint girth can be measured by taking a circumferential measurement with a tape measure around the ankle joint line.

The ankle joint line can be recognized by identifying three points around the ankle. Firstly, mark 1.5 cm above the medial malleolus of the tibia. Secondly, mark 2 cm above the lateral malleolus of the fibula.

Owing to the possibility of a different length or bony changes to the tips of either malleoli, a third point to aid in the triangulation of all the points is identified. The clinician runs their thumb down the anterior border of the tibia until they feel their thumb fall into the dip of the ankle, the anterior joint line.

To confirm this position the clinician can move the ankle joint through plantarflexion and dorsiflexion and feel the talus move against the thumb. This enables confirmation of the anterior joint line of the ankle.

The joint is encircled with a tape measure around the joint line. The circumferential measurement is then recorded.

Repeat the procedure three times and produce an average reading.

Repeat the procedure on the other limb to compare the joint girth.

Points to note:
   The state of the tape measure – is it stretched?
   The muscles must be relaxed.
   Keep the tape measure straight (not twisted).
   Measure consistently – at the top/bottom of the tape, and either in centimetres or in inches.

THE ANKLE JOINT

Notes

Treatment record

LIMB GIRTH
Calf

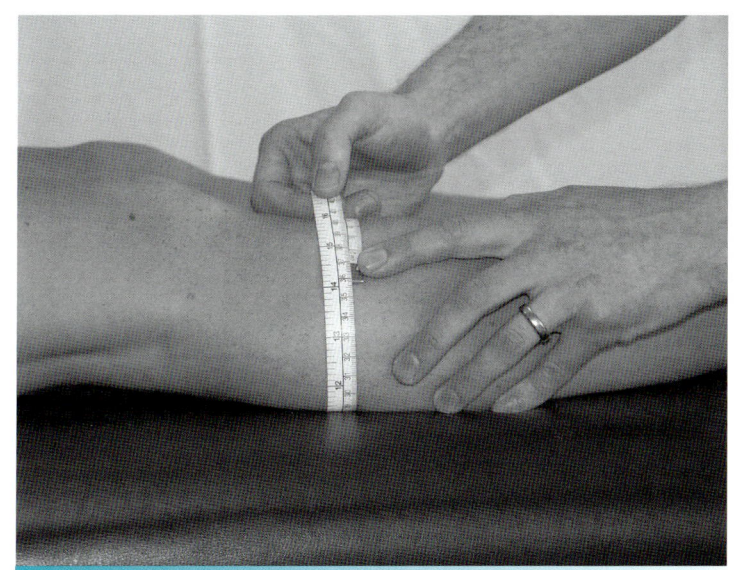

Fig 3.7 Measurement of the girth of the calf.

Patient's position: The patient is positioned in long sitting or half lying on the plinth, well supported. The knees are in passive extension so that the calf and thigh muscles are relaxed.

Method: Mark two or three points – 5 cm (2 inches), 10 cm (4 inches) and 15 cm (6 inches) below the distal end of the tibial tuberosity. (If the patient is small in stature, the measure at 15 cm (6 inches) may not be necessary.)

The limb is encircled with a tape measure at each marked point. The circumferential measurements are then recorded. Repeat the procedure three times and produce an average reading. Repeat the procedure on the other limb to compare the measurements.

Points to note:
  The state of the tape measure – is it stretched?
  The muscles must be relaxed.
  Keep the tape measure straight (not twisted).
  Measure consistently – at the top/bottom of the tape, and either in centimetres or in inches.

THE ANKLE JOINT

Notes

Treatment record

MUSCLE STRENGTH: OXFORD MUSCLE GRADING

Plantarflexors

Grade 0 – 'No contraction' and Grade 1 – 'Flicker of a contraction'

Patient's position: The patient is positioned in prone lying on the plinth, their feet resting over the end of the plinth.

Clinician's position: The clinician is standing at the foot of the plinth with both hands palpating the gastrocnemius muscle for a contraction.

Command to patient: 'Try and tighten your calf muscles/try and move your foot up towards the ceiling.'

Clinical tip: Closely observing and feeling the muscle is essential in enabling the clinician to pick up on even the smallest flicker of a contraction.

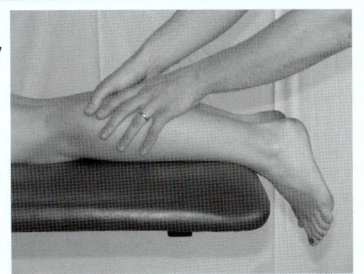

Fig 3.8 Oxford muscle grading for the ankle plantarflexors – Grades 0 and 1.

Grade 2 – 'Full ROM with the effects of gravity eliminated'

Patient's position: The patient is positioned in side lying on the plinth. Their foot is supported in full dorsiflexion.

Clinician's position: The clinician is standing by the patient, supporting the limb with one hand just below the knee and the other supporting the foot.

Command to patient: 'Try and push your foot away from your leg as far as you can.'

The ankle has to move through its full range of movement – full dorsiflexion to full plantarflexion.

Clinical tip: The limb can be heavy, so the safe positioning of the clinician is an essential part of this measurement technique.

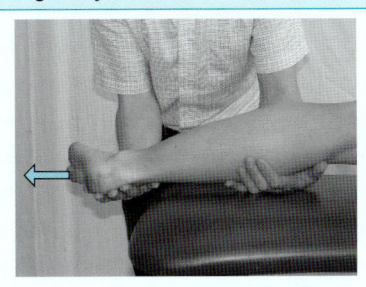

Fig 3.9 Oxford muscle grading for the ankle plantarflexors – Grade 2. The ankle is moving from full dorsiflexion to full plantarflexion.

THE ANKLE JOINT

Grade 3 – 'Full ROM against the effects of gravity'

Patient's position: The patient is positioned in prone lying, with their feet over the end of the plinth. The foot is in full dorsiflexion.

Clinician's position: The clinician is standing at the foot of the plinth to observe the movement.

Command to patient: 'Move your foot upwards towards the ceiling as far as you can.'

The ankle has to move through its full range of movement – full dorsiflexion to full plantarflexion.

Clinical tip: Make sure the patient is in a fully plantarflexed position with the anterior tibial muscles (tibialis anterior, extensor digitorum longus, extensor hallucis longus) relaxed. This can be achieved by palpating the anterior tibial muscles to assess muscle activity.

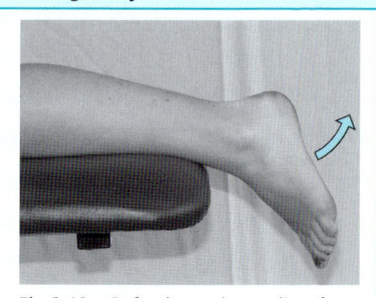

Fig 3.10 Oxford muscle grading for the ankle plantarflexors – Grade 3. The ankle is moving from full dorsiflexion to full plantarflexion (the sole of the foot is moving upwards).

Grade 4 – 'Full ROM against minimal resistance'

Patient's position: The patient is positioned in prone lying, with their feet over the end of the plinth. Their foot is in full dorsiflexion.

Clinician's position: The clinician is standing at the foot of the plinth, applying a minimal resistance to the patient's foot.

Command to patient: 'Push your foot up as far as you can against the minimal resistance.'

The ankle has to move through its full range of movement – full dorsiflexion to full plantarflexion.

Clinical tip: Use the length of lever arm principle to make sure you can apply a consistent resistance to the limb. Ask the patient to start slowly so they can appreciate the amount of resistance.

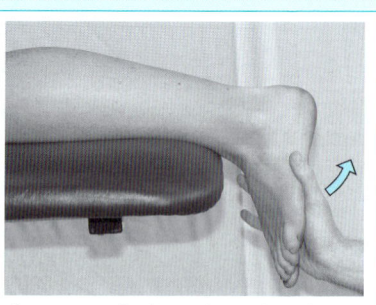

Fig 3.11 Oxford muscle grading for the ankle plantarflexors – Grades 4 and 5. The ankle is moving from full dorsiflexion to full plantarflexion (the sole of the foot is moving upwards).

Grade 5 – 'Full ROM against maximal resistance'

Patient's position: The patient is positioned in prone lying, with their feet over the end of the plinth (see Fig. 3.11).

Clinician's position: The clinician is standing at the foot of the plinth, applying a maximal resistance to the patient's lower leg.

Command to patient: 'Push your foot up as far as you can against the maximal resistance.'

The ankle has to move through its full range of movement – full dorsiflexion to full plantarflexion.

Clinical tip: Use the length of lever arm principle to make sure you can apply a consistent resistance to the limb. Ask the patient to start slowly so they can appreciate the amount of resistance. Remember, the patient's calf muscles may be stronger than your applied resistance; use a safe and mechanically advantageous position to enable you to perform this technique safely and effectively.

Dorsiflexors

Grade 0 – 'No contraction' and Grade 1 – 'Flicker of a contraction'

Patient's position: The patient is positioned in prone lying or long sitting on the plinth, their feet over the end of the plinth.

Clinician's position: The clinician is standing at the foot of the plinth, with both hands palpating the tibialis anterior muscle for a contraction

Command to patient: 'Try and tighten the muscles on the front of your leg/pull your foot up towards you.'

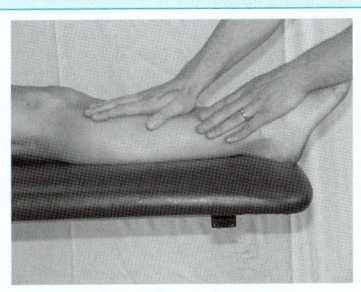

Fig 3.12 Oxford muscle grading for the ankle dorsiflexors – Grades 0 and 1.

Clinical tip: Closely observing and feeling the muscle is essential in enabling the clinician to pick up on even the smallest flicker of a contraction.

Tibialis anterior is a prominent muscle on the anterior aspect of the leg. The tendon is the most medial of the tendons at the front of the ankle joint.

THE ANKLE JOINT

Grade 2 – 'Full ROM with the effects of gravity eliminated'

Patient's position: The patient is positioned in side lying on the plinth. The foot is supported in full plantarflexion.

Clinician's position: The clinician is standing by the patient, supporting the right limb with one hand under the knee area and the other supporting the foot.

Command to patient: 'Try and pull your foot up as far as you can.'

The ankle has to move through its full range of movement – full plantarflexion to full dorsiflexion.

Clinical tip: The limb can be heavy, so the safe positioning of the clinician is an essential part of this measurement technique.

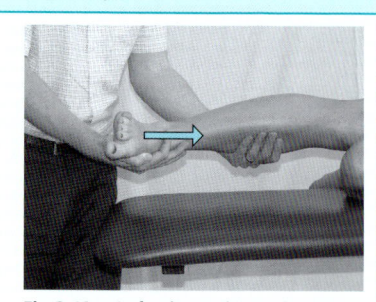

Fig 3.13 Oxford muscle grading for the ankle dorsiflexors – Grade 2. The ankle is moving from full plantarflexion to full dorsiflexion (the dorsum of the foot is moving towards the shin).

Grade 3 – 'Full ROM against the effects of gravity'

Patient's position: The patient is positioned in supine lying or long sitting on the plinth. Their foot is hanging over the end of the plinth in full plantarflexion.

Clinician's position: The clinician is standing at the foot of the plinth to observe the movement.

Command to patient: 'Pull your foot upwards as far as you can.'

The ankle has to move through its full range of movement – full plantarflexion to full dorsiflexion.

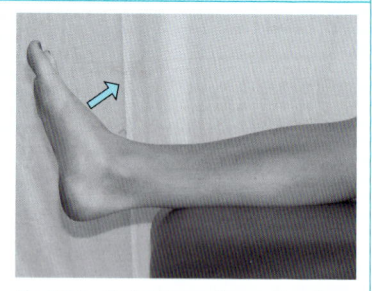

Fig 3.14 Oxford muscle grading for the ankle dorsiflexors – Grade 3. The ankle is moving from full plantarflexion to full dorsiflexion (the dorsum of the foot is moving up towards the shin).

Grade 4 – 'Full ROM against minimal resistance'

Patient's position: The patient is positioned in supine lying or long sitting on the plinth. Their foot is hanging over the end of the plinth in full plantarflexion.

Clinician's position: The clinician is standing at the foot of the plinth, applying a minimal resistance to the top of the patient's foot.

Command to patient: 'Push your foot up as far as you can against the minimal resistance.'

The ankle has to move through its full range of movement – full plantarflexion to full dorsiflexion.

Clinical tip: Use the length of lever arm principle to make sure you can apply a consistent resistance to the limb. Ask the patient to start slowly so they can appreciate the amount of resistance.

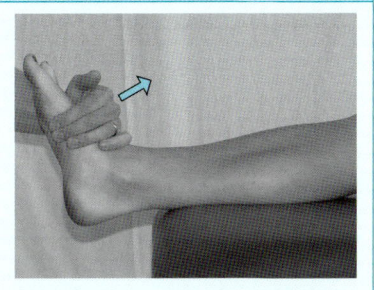

Fig 3.15 Oxford muscle grading for the ankle dorsiflexors – Grades 4 and 5. The ankle is moving from full plantarflexion to full dorsiflexion (the dorsum of the foot is moving up towards the shin).

Grade 5 – 'Full ROM against maximal resistance'

Patient's position: The patient is positioned in supine lying or long sitting on the plinth. Their foot is hanging over the end of the plinth in full plantarflexion (see Fig. 3.15).

Clinician's position: The clinician is standing at the foot of the plinth, applying a maximal resistance to the patient's lower leg.

Command to patient: 'Push your foot up as far as you can against the maximal resistance.'

The ankle has to move through its full range of movement – full plantarflexion to full dorsiflexion.

Clinical tip: Use the length of lever arm principle to make sure you can apply a consistent resistance to the limb. Ask the patient to start slowly so they can appreciate the amount of resistance. Remember, the patient's anterior tibial muscles may be stronger than your applied resistance. You must use a safe and mechanically advantageous position to enable you to perform this technique safely and effectively.

THE ANKLE JOINT

Evertors

Grade 0 – 'No contraction' and Grade 1 – 'Flicker of a contraction'

Patient's position: The patient is positioned in long sitting on the plinth, with their foot over the end of the plinth.

Clinician's position: The clinician is standing at the foot of the plinth with both hands palpating the lateral aspect of the leg, over the peroneal muscles (peroneus longus and brevis).

Command to patient: 'Try and turn your foot outwards (by using the muscles on the side of your leg).'

Clinical tip: Closely observing and feeling the muscles is essential in enabling the clinician to pick up on even the smallest flicker of a contraction.

Peroneus longus and brevis can be felt to contract on the lateral side of the leg, below the head of the fibula. The tendons can be palpated as they pass behind the lateral malleolus of the fibula.

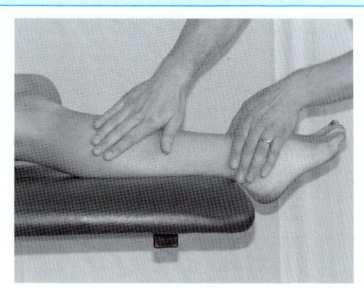

Fig 3.16 Oxford muscle grading for the ankle evertors – Grades 0 and 1.

Grade 2 – 'Full ROM with the effects of gravity eliminated'

Patient's position: The patient is positioned in supine lying or long sitting on the plinth, their inverted foot over the end of the plinth.

Clinician's position: The clinician is standing at the foot of the plinth, supporting the calcaneus and the foot.

Command to patient: 'Try and turn your foot outwards as far as you can.'

The ankle has to move through its full range of movement – full inversion to full eversion.

Clinical tip: The leg and foot can be heavy, so the safe positioning of the clinician is an essential part of this measurement technique. This has to be balanced against being able to take the weight of the foot, but not actually assisting the patient's efforts to evert the foot.

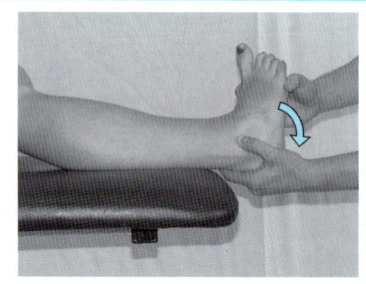

Fig 3.17 Oxford muscle grading for the ankle evertors – Grade 2. The ankle is moving from full inversion to full eversion (the foot is moving from being fully turned in to being fully turned out).

Grade 3 – 'Full ROM against the effects of gravity'

Patient's position: The patient is positioned in side lying on the plinth, their inverted foot over the end of the plinth.

Clinician's position: The clinician is standing at the foot of the plinth to observe the movement.

Command to patient: 'Try and turn the sole of your foot so that it is facing towards the ceiling.'

The ankle has to move through its full range of movement – full inversion to full eversion.

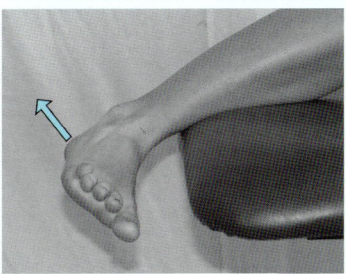

Fig 3.18 Oxford muscle grading for the ankle evertors – Grade 3. The ankle is moving from full inversion to full eversion (the sole of the foot is turning up towards the ceiling).

Grade 4 – 'Full ROM against minimal resistance'

Patient's position: The patient is positioned in side lying on the plinth, their inverted foot over the end of the plinth.

Clinician's position: The clinician is standing at the foot of the plinth, applying a minimal resistance to the lateral border of the foot.

Command to patient: 'Try and turn the sole of your foot so that it is facing towards the ceiling against the minimal resistance.'

The ankle has to move through its full range of movement – full inversion to full eversion.

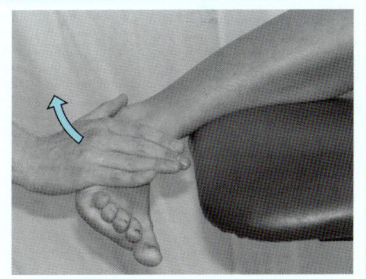

Fig 3.19 Oxford muscle grading for the ankle evertors – Grades 4 and 5. The ankle is moving from full inversion to full eversion (the sole of the foot is turning up towards the ceiling).

Grade 5 – 'Full ROM against maximal resistance'

Patient's position: The patient is positioned in side lying on the plinth, their inverted foot over the end of the plinth (see Fig. 3.19).

Clinician's position: The clinician is standing at the foot of the plinth, applying a maximal resistance to the lateral border of the foot.

Command to patient: 'Try and turn the sole of your foot so that it is facing towards the ceiling against the maximal resistance.'

The ankle has to move through its full range of movement – full inversion to full eversion.

THE ANKLE JOINT

Invertors

Grade 0 – 'No contraction' and Grade 1 – 'Flicker of a contraction'

Patient's position: The patient is positioned in long sitting on the plinth, their everted foot over the end of the plinth.

Clinician's position: The clinician is standing at the foot of the plinth with their hand palpating the tendon of tibialis posterior on the medial aspect of the ankle joint.

Command to patient: 'Try and turn your foot inwards by using the muscles on the inside of your leg.'

Clinical tip: Closely observing and feeling the tendon is essential in enabling the clinician to pick up on even the smallest flicker of a contraction. Tibialis posterior is a deep calf muscle, but it can be palpated behind the medial malleolus of the tibia.

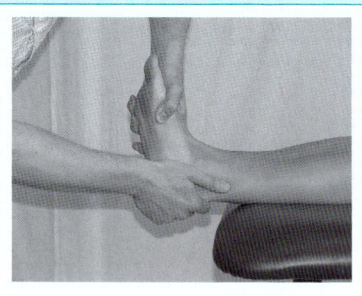

Fig 3.20 Oxford muscle grading for the ankle invertors – Grades 0 and 1.

Grade 2 – 'Full ROM with the effects of gravity eliminated'

Patient's position: The patient is positioned in supine lying or long sitting on the plinth, their everted foot over the end of the plinth.

Clinician's position: The clinician is standing at the foot of the plinth, supporting the calcaneus and the foot.

Command to patient: 'Try and turn your foot inwards as far as you can.'

The ankle has to move through its full range of movement – full eversion to full inversion.

Clinical tip: The foot can be heavy, so the safe positioning of the clinician is an essential part of this measurement technique. This has to be balanced against being able to take the weight of the foot, but not actually assisting the patient's efforts to invert the foot.

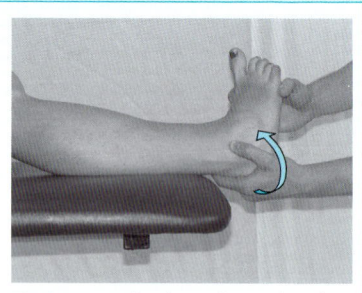

Fig 3.21 Oxford muscle grading for the ankle invertors – Grade 2. The ankle has moved from full inversion to full eversion (the foot has moved from being fully turned out to being fully turned in).

Measurement

Grade 3 – 'Full ROM against the effects of gravity'

Patient's position: The patient is positioned in side lying on the plinth, their everted foot over the end of the plinth.

Clinician's position: The clinician is standing at the foot of the plinth observing the movement.

Command to patient: 'Try and turn the sole of your foot so that it is facing towards the ceiling.'

The ankle has to move through its full range of movement – full eversion to full inversion.

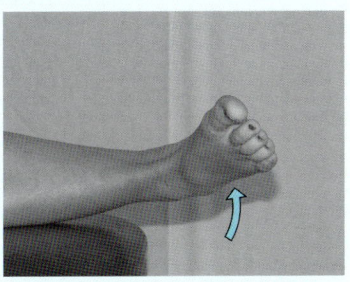

Fig 3.22 Oxford muscle grading for the ankle invertors – Grade 3. The ankle has moved from full eversion to full inversion (the foot has moved from being fully turned out to being fully turned in).

Grade 4 – 'Full ROM against minimal resistance'

Patient's position: The patient is positioned in side lying on the plinth, their everted foot over the end of the plinth.

Clinician's position: The clinician is standing at the foot of the plinth, applying a minimal resistance to the medial border of the foot.

Command to patient: 'Try and turn the sole of your foot so that it is facing towards the ceiling against the minimal resistance.'

The ankle has to move through its full range of movement – full eversion to full inversion.

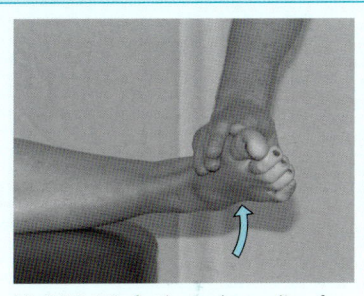

Fig 3.23 Oxford muscle grading for the ankle invertors – Grades 4 and 5. The ankle has moved from full eversion to full inversion (the foot has moved from being fully turned out to being fully turned in).

> ### Grade 5 – 'Full ROM against maximal resistance'
>
> **Patient's position:** The patient is positioned in side lying on the plinth, their everted foot over the end of the plinth (see Fig. 3.23).
>
> **Clinician's position:** The clinician is standing at the foot of the plinth, applying a maximal resistance to the medial border of the foot.
>
> **Command to patient:** 'Try and turn the sole of your foot so that it is facing towards the ceiling against the maximal resistance.'
>
> The ankle has to move through its full range of movement – full eversion to full inversion.

Measurement

Notes

Treatment record

THE ANKLE JOINT

Notes

Treatment record

CHAPTER 4

The shoulder joint

ANATOMY 89
   Bony landmarks to be palpated 90
   Ligaments 90
   Muscles 91
      Flexors 91
      Extensors 92
      Adductors 93
      Abductors 94
      Lateral (external) rotators 94
      Medial (internal) rotators 95
MEASUREMENT 96
   Range of movement 96
      Extension 96
      Flexion 97
      Abduction 98
      Adduction 99
      Medial (internal) rotation 100
      Lateral (external) rotation 101
      Observational/reflective checklist 103
   Limb girth 104
      Upper limb 104
      Observational/reflective checklist 106
   Muscle strength: Oxford muscle grading 107
      Flexors 107
      Extensors 109
      Abductors 112
      Adductors 114
      Medial (internal) rotators 117
      Lateral (external) rotators 120

ANATOMY

1. The shoulder joint is a synovial ball and socket joint.
2. It is the articulation between the head of the humerus (ball) and the glenoid fossa (socket) of the scapula.
3. It has a loose capsule surrounding the joint, allowing for the large range of movement and multiple degrees of freedom associated with this joint. There is an increased laxity in the capsule inferiorly, to allow for abduction at the joint.
4. The joint is strengthened anteriorly by capsular ligaments (superior, middle and inferior glenohumeral ligaments).

5. The joint is also strengthened by the rotator cuff muscles – supraspinatus, infraspinatus, teres minor and subscapularis.
6. The glenoid fossa is deepened by the glenoid labrum, a thick wedge of cartilage that surrounds the articular margins, increasing the congruency of the joint.
7. The movements that take place at the shoulder joint are: flexion, extension, abduction, adduction, lateral (external) rotation and medial (internal) rotation.

BONY LANDMARKS TO BE PALPATED

The scapula – acromion process, acromion angle, spine of the scapula, coracoid process, inferior angle and medial border.

The humerus – greater tubercle, lesser tubercle and the intertubercular groove.

LIGAMENTS

Table 4.1

The ligaments of the shoulder

Ligament	Origin	Insertion	Limitations to movement
Superior glenohumeral	Upper part of the glenoid margin and adjacent labrum of the scapula	Upper surface of the lesser tubercle of the humerus	Lateral rotation
Middle glenohumeral	Middle part of the glenoid margin and adjacent labrum of the scapula	Lesser tubercle of the humerus	Lateral rotation
Inferior glenohumeral	Lower aspect of the glenoid margin and adjacent labrum of the scapula	Anteroinferior aspect of the anatomical neck of the humerus	Lateral rotation and possible limitation of abduction in its outer range
Transverse humeral	Greater tubercle of the humerus	Lesser tubercle of the humerus	Bridges the gap between the two tubercles, thus holding the long head of biceps tendon in the intertubercular groove
Coracohumeral	Coracoid process of the scapula	Anterior part of the ligament attaches to the lesser tubercle Posterior part attaches to the greater tubercle of the humerus	Blends with the capsule to enhance the capsular strength
Coracoacromial	Lateral border of the coracoid process of the scapula	Anterior aspect of the acromion of the scapula, in front of the acromioclavicular joint	Limits upward migration of the humerus

MUSCLES
Flexors

Table 4.2

The flexors of the shoulder

Muscle	Origin	Insertion	Nerve supply	Action(s)
Pectoralis major	Medial half of the anterior surface of the clavicle and the lateral aspect of the body of the sternum	Into the lateral lip of the intertubercular groove of the humerus	Medial C8 and lateral C5, 6, 7 pectoral nerves	Medial rotation and adduction of the shoulder joint Clavicular part = shoulder flexion Sternal part = shoulder extension from a flexed position
Deltoid	Anterior fibres = lateral third of the anterior aspect of the clavicle Middle fibres = lateral aspect of the acromion of the scapula Posterior fibres = lateral third of the lower aspect of the spine of the scapula	Deltoid tuberosity of the humerus	Axillary nerve C5, 6	Anterior fibres = flexion of the shoulder Middle fibres = abduction of the shoulder Posterior fibres = extension of the shoulder
Coracobrachialis	Coracoid process of the scapula	Medial side of the shaft of the humerus, approximately a third of the way down the shaft	Musculocutaneous nerve C6, 7	Flexion and adduction of the shoulder joint
Biceps brachii (long head)	Long head = superior glenoid tubercle of the scapula Short head = coracoid process of the scapula	Bicipital aponeurosis and the radial tuberosity	Musculocutaneous nerve C5, 6	Long head = flexion of the shoulder joint Long head and short head = flexion and supination of the elbow

Extensors

Table 4.3

The extensors of the shoulder				
Muscle	Origin	Insertion	Nerve supply	Action(s)
Pectoralis major	Medial half of the anterior surface of the clavicle and the lateral aspect of the body of the sternum	Into the lateral lip of the intertubercular groove of the humerus	Medial C8 and lateral C5, 6, 7 pectoral nerves	Medial rotation and adduction of the shoulder joint Clavicular part = shoulder flexion Sternal part = shoulder extension from a flexed position
Deltoid	Anterior fibres = lateral third of the anterior aspect of the clavicle Middle fibres = lateral aspect of the acromion of the scapula Posterior fibres = lateral third of the lower aspect of the spine of the scapula	Deltoid tuberosity of the humerus	Axillary nerve C5, 6	Anterior fibres = flexion of the shoulder Middle fibres = abduction of the shoulder Posterior fibres = extension of the shoulder
Latissimus dorsi	Lateral aspects of the thoracolumbar fascia, which is in turn attached to the spinous process and the ligamentous attachments of the lower six thoracic vertebrae and all five lumbar vertebrae, also the sacrum. The outer lip of the distal third of the iliac crest, the outer surface of the lower three or four ribs and the inferior angle of scapula	Intertubercular groove of the humerus	Thoracodorsal nerve C6, 7, 8	Extension (of the flexed arm), adduction and medial rotation of the humerus
Teres major	Lower quarter of the lateral border and dorsal surface of the inferior angle of the scapula	Medial lip of the intertubercular groove on the humerus	Lower subscapular nerve C6, 7	Extension of the flexed arm, adduction and medial rotation of the humerus
Triceps brachii	Lateral head = above the spiral groove on the posterior surface of the humerus Long head = infraglenoid tubercle of the scapula Medial head = below the spiral groove on the medial aspect of the posterior surface of the humerus	Posterior part of the olecranon of the ulna	Radial nerve C6, 7, 8	Extension of the shoulder from a flexed position, adduction of the shoulder joint and extension of the elbow

Adductors

Table 4.4

| The adductors of the shoulder |||||
Muscle	Origin	Insertion	Nerve supply	Action(s)
Pectoralis major	Medial half of the anterior surface of the clavicle and the lateral aspect of the body of the sternum	Into the lateral lip of the intertubercular groove of the humerus	Medial C8 and lateral C5, 6, 7 pectoral nerves	Medial rotation and adduction of the shoulder Clavicular part = flexion of the shoulder Sternal part = shoulder extension from a flexed position
Latissimus dorsi	Lateral aspects of the thoracolumbar fascia, which is in turn attached to the spinous process and the ligamentous attachments of the lower six thoracic vertebrae and all five lumbar vertebrae, also the sacrum. The outer lip of the distal third of the iliac crest, the outer surface of the lower three or four ribs and the inferior angle of scapula	Intertubercular groove of the humerus	Thoracodorsal nerve C6, 7, 8	Extension (of the flexed arm), adduction and medial rotation of the humerus
Teres major	Lower quarter of the lateral border and dorsal surface of the inferior angle of the scapula	Medial lip of the intertubercular groove on the humerus	Lower subscapular nerve C6, 7	Extension of the flexed arm, adduction and medial rotation of the humerus
Coraco-brachialis	Coracoid process of the scapula	Medial side of the shaft of the humerus, approximately a third of the way down the shaft	Musculo-cutaneous nerve C6, 7	Flexion and adduction of the shoulder joint

Abductors

Table 4.5

The abductors of the shoulder

Muscle	Origin	Insertion	Nerve supply	Action(s)
Deltoid	Anterior fibres = lateral third of the anterior aspect of the clavicle Middle fibres = lateral aspect of the acromion of the scapula Posterior fibres = lateral third of the lower aspect of the spine of the scapula	Deltoid tuberosity of the humerus	Axillary nerve C5, 6	Anterior fibres = flexion of the shoulder Middle fibres = abduction of the shoulder Posterior fibres = extension of the shoulder
Supraspinatus	Medial two-thirds of the supraspinous fossa of the scapula	Greater tubercle (upper facet) on the humerus	Suprascapular nerve C5, 6	Abduction of the shoulder joint, and a stabilizer of the shoulder joint

Lateral (external) rotators

Table 4.6

The lateral (external) rotators of the shoulder

Muscle	Origin	Insertion	Nerve supply	Action(s)
Deltoid	Anterior fibres = lateral third of the anterior aspect of the clavicle Middle fibres = lateral aspect of the acromion of the scapula Posterior fibres = lateral third of the lower aspect of the spine of the scapula	Deltoid tuberosity of the humerus	Axillary nerve C5, 6	Anterior fibres = flexion of the shoulder Middle fibres = abduction of the shoulder Posterior fibres = extension and lateral rotation of the shoulder
Infraspinatus	Medial two-thirds of the infraspinous fossa of the scapula	Greater tubercle (middle facet) on the humerus	Suprascapular nerve C5, 6	Lateral rotation and stabilizer of the shoulder joint
Teres minor	Upper two-thirds of the lateral border of the scapula	Greater tubercle (inferior facet) on the humerus	Axillary nerve C5, 6	Lateral rotation and adduction from an abducted humerus

Anatomy

Medial (internal) rotators

Table 4.7

The medial (internal) rotators of the shoulder

Muscle	Origin	Insertion	Nerve supply	Action(s)
Deltoid	Anterior fibres = lateral third of the anterior aspect of the clavicle Middle fibres = lateral aspect of the acromion of the scapula Posterior fibres = lateral third of the lower aspect of the spine of the scapula	Deltoid tuberosity of the humerus	Axillary nerve C5, 6	Anterior fibres = flexion and medial rotation of the shoulder Middle fibres = abduction of the shoulder Posterior fibres = extension of the shoulder
Sub-scapularis	Medial two-thirds of the subscapular fossa on the scapular	Lesser tubercle of the humerus	Subscapular nerve C5, 6, 7	Medial rotation and adduction of the shoulder joint
Teres major	Lower quarter of the lateral border and dorsal surface of the inferior angle of the scapula	Medial lip of the intertubercular groove on the humerus	Lower subscapular nerve C6, 7	Extension of the flexed arm, adduction and medial rotation of the humerus
Latissimus dorsi	Lateral aspects of the thoracolumbar fascia, which is in turn attached to the spinous process and the ligamentous attachments of the lower six thoracic vertebrae and all five lumbar vertebrae, also the sacrum. The outer lip of the distal third of the iliac crest, the outer surface of the lower three or four ribs and the inferior angle of the scapula	Intertubercular groove of the humerus	Thoracodorsal nerve C6, 7, 8	Extension (of the flexed arm), adduction and medial rotation of the humerus
Pectoralis major	Medial half of the anterior surface of the clavicle and the lateral aspect of the body of the sternum	Into the lateral lip of the intertubercular groove of the humerus	Medial C8 and lateral C5, 6, 7 pectoral nerves	Medial rotation, adduction of the shoulder Clavicular part = shoulder flexion Sternal part = shoulder extension from a flexed position

THE SHOULDER JOINT

MEASUREMENT

RANGE OF MOVEMENT
Extension

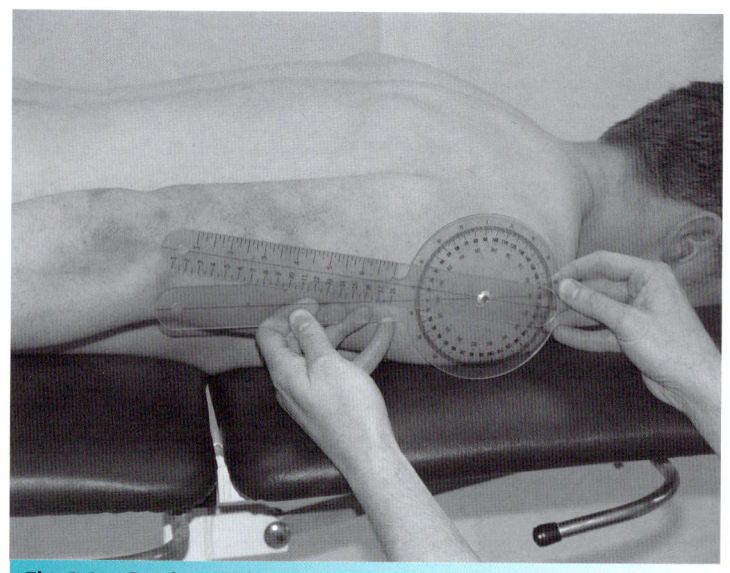

Fig 4.1 Goniometric measurement of shoulder extension.

Starting position: The patient is positioned in prone lying on the plinth (or sitting), their arm resting at the side, palm facing medially.
Goniometer axis: The axis of the goniometer is placed over the lateral aspect of the centre of the humeral head, approximately 2.5 cm inferior to the lateral aspect of acromial process.
Stationary arm: This is parallel to lateral mid-line of the trunk.
Moveable arm: This is parallel to longitudinal axis of the humerus, pointing towards the lateral epicondyle of the humerus.
Command to patient: 'Keeping your elbow straight, move your arm backwards, as far as you can.'
End position: The humerus moves posteriorly, to the limit of motion.
Trick movements: Scapular anterior tilting, elevation and shoulder abduction. The patient may also flex the trunk.

NB: It may be necessary to reposition the stationary and moveable arms of the goniometer prior to taking the reading, as they may have moved when the patient extended their shoulder.

Flexion

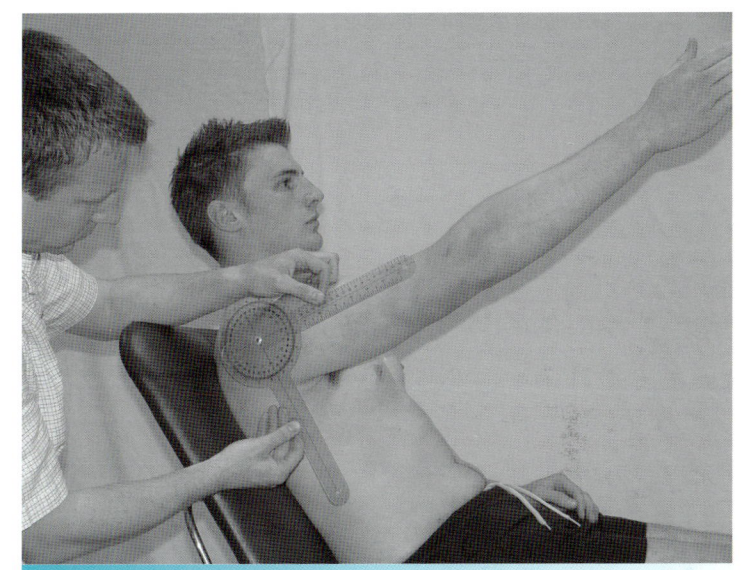

Fig 4.2 Goniometric measurement of shoulder flexion.

Starting position: The patient is positioned in half lying on the plinth or sitting, their arm at their side, palm facing medially.
Goniometer axis: The axis of the goniometer is placed over the lateral aspect of the centre of the humeral head, approximately 2.5 cm inferior to the lateral aspect of acromial process.
Stationary arm: This is parallel to the mid-line of the trunk.
Moveable arm: This is parallel to the longitudinal axis of the humerus, pointing towards the lateral epicondyle of the humerus.
Command to patient: 'Keeping your elbow straight, move your arm forwards and upwards as far as you can.'
End position: The humerus moves in an anterior direction to the limit of motion.

NB: It may be necessary to reposition the stationary and moveable arms of the goniometer prior to taking the reading, as they may have moved when the patient flexed their shoulder.

THE SHOULDER JOINT

Abduction

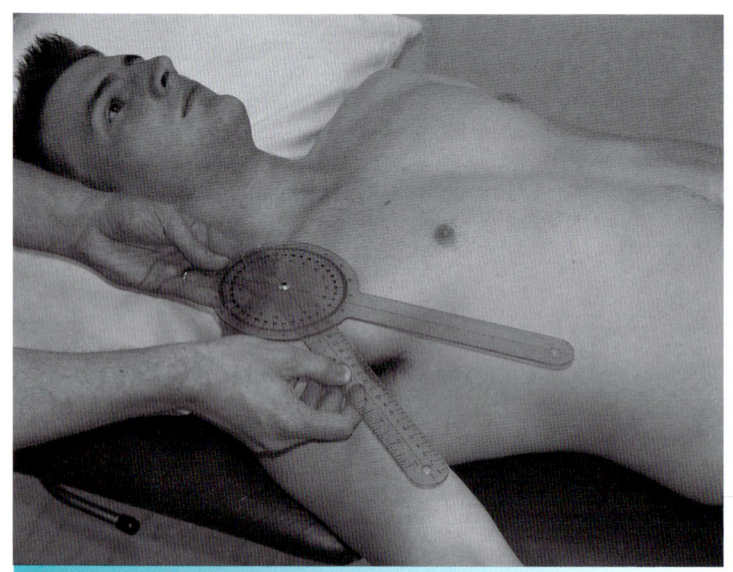

Fig 4.3 Goniometric measurement of shoulder abduction.

Starting position: The patient is positioned in supine lying on the plinth or sitting, their arm at their side, palm facing medially.
Goniometer axis: The axis of the goniometer is placed over the mid-point of the anterior aspect of the glenohumeral joint, approximately 1.5 cm inferior and lateral to the coracoid process of the scapula.
Stationary arm: This is parallel to the mid-sternal line.
Moveable arm: This is parallel to the longitudinal axis of the humerus, pointing towards the lateral epicondyle of the humerus.
Command to patient: 'Move your arm outwards and upwards towards your head as far as you can, keeping your palm facing the same way.'
End position: The humerus moves laterally to the limit of motion.
Trick movements: Contralateral trunk side flexion, scapular elevation, and shoulder flexion.

Adduction

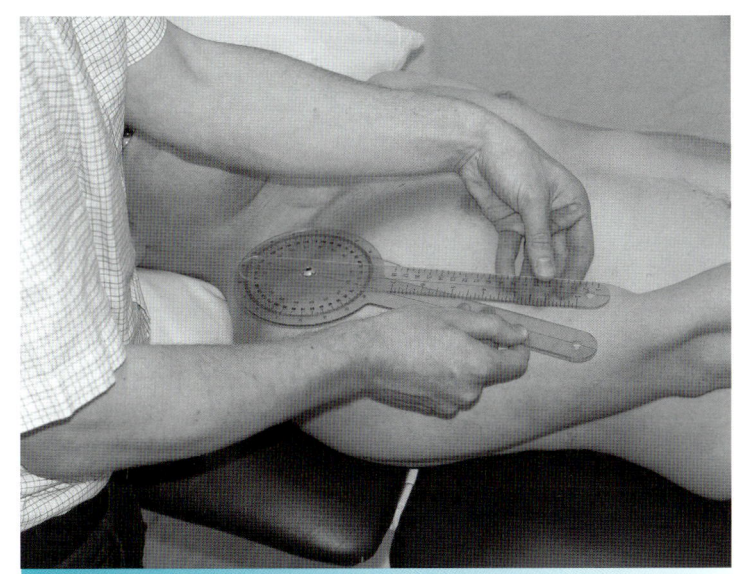

Fig 4.4 Goniometric measurement of shoulder adduction.

Starting position The patient is positioned in supine lying on the plinth or sitting, their arm at their side, palm facing medially.
Goniometer axis: The axis of the goniometer is placed over the mid-point of the anterior aspect of the glenohumeral joint, approximately 1.5 cm inferior and lateral to the coracoid process.
Stationary arm: This is parallel to the mid-sternal line.
Moveable arm: This is parallel to the longitudinal axis of the humerus, pointing towards the lateral epicondyle of the humerus.
Command to patient: 'Move your arm across your body, as far as you can towards the opposite side of the plinth.'
End position: The humerus moves medially to the limit of motion.

Clinical tip
The shoulder has to be in some degree of flexion to achieve shoulder adduction.

Medial (internal) rotation

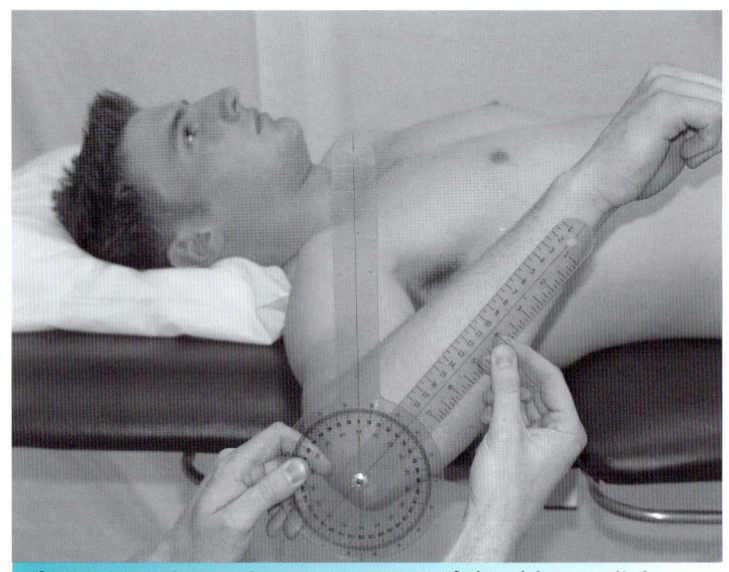

Fig 4.5 Goniometric measurement of shoulder medial (internal) rotation.

Starting position: The patient is positioned in supine lying on the plinth, their shoulder in 90° of abduction, the elbow flexed to 90° and the forearm in the pronated position. A towel is placed under the humerus to achieve an abducted position.
Goniometer axis: The axis of the goniometer is placed on the olecranon process of the ulna.
Stationary arm: This is perpendicular to the floor.
Moveable arm: This is parallel to the longitudinal axis of the ulna, pointing towards the ulnar styloid process.
Command to patient: 'Move your palm downwards towards the floor.'
End position: The palm of the hand is moved towards the floor to the limit of medial rotation.
Trick movements: Elbow extension, scapular elevation and abduction.

Lateral (external) rotation

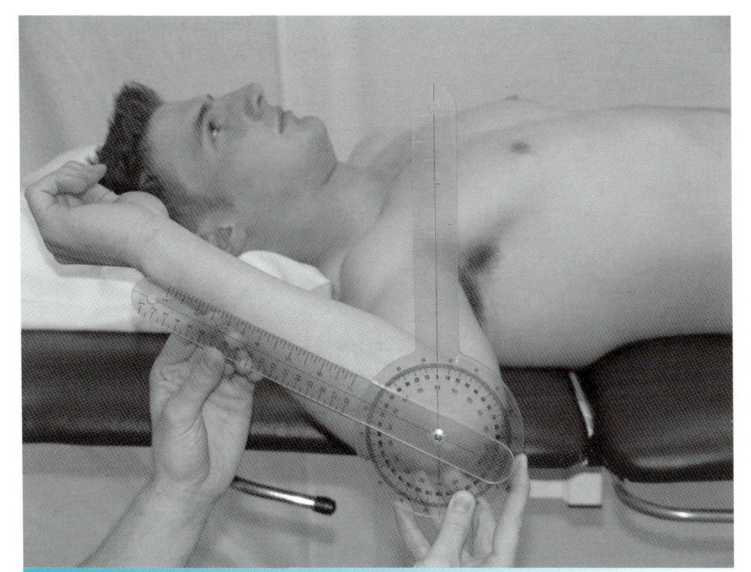

Fig 4.6 Goniometric measurement of shoulder lateral (external) rotation.

Starting position: The patient is positioned in supine lying, their shoulder in 90° of abduction, the elbow flexed to 90° and the forearm in the pronated position. A folded towel is placed under the humerus.
Goniometer axis: The axis of the goniometer is placed on the olecranon.
Stationary arm: This is perpendicular to the trunk.
Moveable arm: This is parallel to the longitudinal axis of the ulna.
Command to patient: 'Move your hand backwards towards the plinth.'
End position: The dorsum of the hand is moved towards the floor to its limit of motion.
Trick movements: Elbow extension, scapular depression, and adduction.

THE SHOULDER JOINT

Notes

Treatment record

Observational/reflective checklist

Observational/ reflective checklist			
Observation		Y/N	Comments
Introduction and preparation for the skill	Was the treatment area properly prepared for the patient, e.g. pillow, blanket, safe environment, etc.?		
	Did the therapist introduce him/herself?		
	Was the patient comfortable?		
	Was the patient adequately exposed/draped?		
	Was an explanation of the procedure given?		
	Was the explanation clear and succinct?		
	Was consent obtained?		
Performing the skill	Was the plinth set at the correct height?		
	Was the therapist's posture compromised?		
	Did the therapist identify the joint and other relevant bony landmarks?		
	Was the goniometer correctly aligned?		
	Was the reading of the joint range of movements accurate?		
	Did the therapist compare both sides of the body?		
Safe and effective performance of the technique	Was the procedure carried out with due care and attention?		
How would you rate the proficiency in the overall performance of the skill?	Excellent		
	Very good		
	Good		
	Satisfactory		
	Borderline		
	Fail		

THE SHOULDER JOINT

LIMB GIRTH
Upper limb

Measurements may need to be taken of the upper limb if, for example, a patient has lymphoedema.

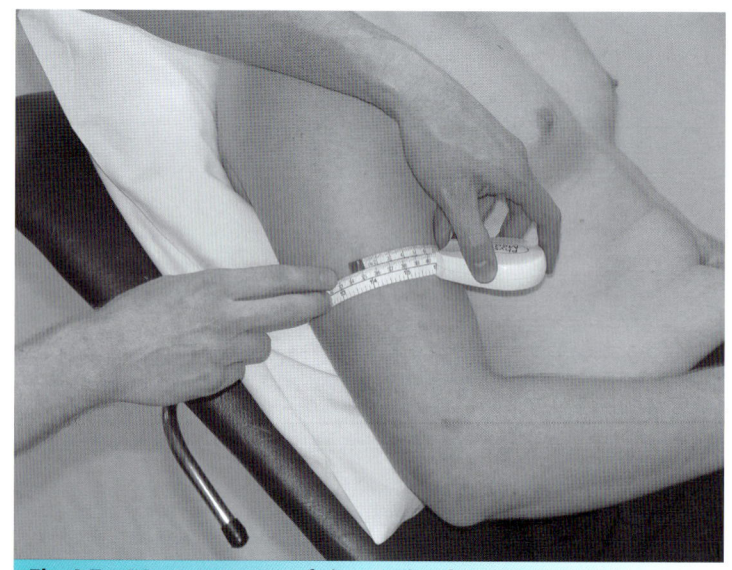

Fig 4.7 Measurement of the girth of the upper limb.

Patient's position: The patient is positioned in long sitting or half lying on the plinth, well supported. Their elbow is resting on a pillow, which is on their lap.
Method: The measurements are taken at 4 cm (1.5 inch) intervals from a fixed point on the olecranon process, with consideration given to the length of the arm and the extent of the swelling. The measurements may therefore extend to the forearm.

The limb is encircled with a tape measure at each marked point. The circumferential measurements are then recorded.

Repeat three times and produce an average reading, then repeat the procedure on the other limb to compare the two.

Points to note:
 The state of the tape measure – is it stretched?
 The muscles must be relaxed.
 Keep the tape measure straight (not twisted).
 Measure consistently – at the top/bottom of the tape, and
   either in centimetres or in inches.

Measurement

Notes

Treatment record

THE SHOULDER JOINT

Observational/reflective checklist

Observational/reflective checklist			
Observation		Y/N	Comments
Introduction and preparation for the skill	Was the treatment area properly prepared for the patient, e.g. pillow, blanket, safe environment, etc.?		
	Did the therapist introduce him/herself?		
	Was the patient comfortable?		
	Was the patient adequately exposed/draped?		
	Was an explanation of the procedure given?		
	Was the explanation clear and succinct?		
	Was consent obtained?		
Performing the skill	Was the plinth set at the correct height?		
	Was the therapist's posture compromised?		
	Did the therapist identify the joint and other relevant bony landmarks?		
	Was the tape measure correctly aligned?		
	Was the reading of the limb girth accurate?		
	Did the therapist compare both sides of the body?		
Safe and effective performance of the technique	Was the procedure carried out with due care and attention?		
How would you rate the proficiency in the overall performance of the skill?	Excellent		
	Very good		
	Good		
	Satisfactory		
	Borderline		
	Fail		

Measurement

MUSCLE STRENGTH: OXFORD MUSCLE GRADING

Flexors

Grade 0 – 'No contraction' and Grade 1 – 'Flicker of a contraction'

Patient's position: The patient is positioned in supine lying on the plinth or in sitting.

Clinician's position: The clinician is standing by the side of the patient, with both hands palpating the anterior deltoid and biceps brachii muscles for a contraction.

Command to patient: 'Try and tighten your shoulder muscles/lift your arm up towards the ceiling.'

Clinical tip: Closely observing and feeling the muscle is essential in enabling the clinician to pick up on even the smallest flicker of a contraction.

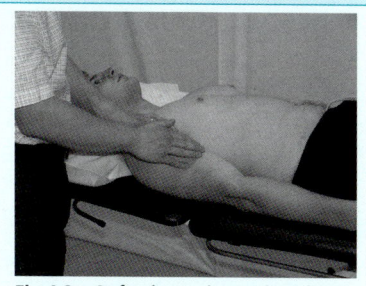

Fig 4.8 Oxford muscle grading for the shoulder flexors – Grades 0 and 1.

Grade 2 – 'Full ROM with the effects of gravity eliminated'

Patient's position: The patient is positioned in side lying on the plinth. The arm is supported in full shoulder extension.

Clinician's position: The clinician is standing by the patient, supporting the limb, with one hand under the elbow and the other just above the wrist.

Command to patient: 'Try and move your arm forwards as far as you can.'

The shoulder has to move through its full range of movement – full extension to full flexion.

Clinical tip: The limb can be heavy, so the safe positioning of the clinician is an essential part of this measurement technique.

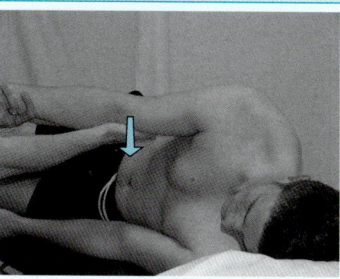

Fig 4.9 Oxford muscle grading for the shoulder flexors – Grade 2. The shoulder is moving from full extension to full flexion (forwards).

THE SHOULDER JOINT

Grade 3 – 'Full ROM against the effects of gravity'

Patient's position: The patient is positioned in standing or sitting, with their arm hanging by their side (neutral). The arm is not starting from full shoulder extension because gravity would be assisting the movement.

Clinician's position: The clinician is standing in front of the patient to observe their movement.

Command to patient: 'Lift your arm forwards as far as you can.'

The shoulder has to move through its full available range of movement – neutral to full flexion.

Clinical tip: Sitting is one of the most suitable positions and easy to progress to testing for Grades 4 and 5.

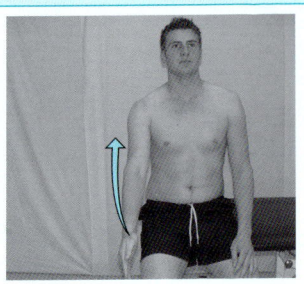

Fig 4.10 Oxford muscle grading for the shoulder flexors – Grade 3. The shoulder is moving from neutral to full flexion (the arm is being raised towards the ceiling).

Grade 4 – 'Full ROM against minimal resistance'

Patient's position: The patient is positioned in standing or sitting, with their arm hanging by their side (neutral). The arm is not starting from full shoulder extension because gravity would be assisting the movement.

Clinician's position: The clinician is standing by the side of the patient, applying a minimal resistance to the distal part of the arm.

Command to patient: 'Lift your arm forwards as far as it will go against the minimal resistance.'

The shoulder has to move through its full available range of movement – neutral to full flexion.

Clinical tip: Use the length of lever arm principle to make sure you can apply a consistent resistance to the limb. Ask the patient to start slowly so they can appreciate the amount of resistance. Also, positioning is essential, as the patient needs to be seated so that you can apply even pressure while they approach full range.

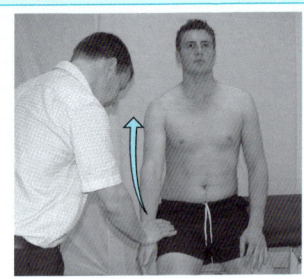

Fig 4.11 Oxford muscle grading for the shoulder flexors – Grades 4 and 5. The shoulder is moving from neutral to full flexion (the arm is being raised towards the ceiling).

Grade 5 – 'Full ROM against maximal resistance'

Patient's position: The patient is positioned in standing or sitting, with their arm hanging by their side (neutral). The arm is not starting from full shoulder extension because gravity would be assisting the movement (see Fig. 4.11).

Clinician's position: The clinician is standing by the side of the patient, applying a maximal resistance to the distal parts of the arm.

Command to patient: 'Lift your arm forwards as far as it will go against the maximal resistance.'

The shoulder has to move through its full available range of movement – neutral to full flexion.

Clinical tip: Remember that maximal resistance is related to the patient's maximum and not your maximal.

Use the length of lever arm principle to make sure you can apply a consistent resistance to the limb. Ask the patient to start slowly so they can appreciate the amount of resistance.

Extensors

Grade 0 – 'No contraction' and Grade 1 – 'Flicker of a contraction'

Patient's position: The patient is positioned in side lying on the plinth.

Clinician's position: The clinician is standing by the patient, with both hands palpating the posterior deltoid muscle for a contraction.

Command to patient: 'Try and tighten your shoulder muscles/try and move your arm backwards.'

Clinical tip: Closely observing and feeling the muscle is essential in enabling the clinician to pick up on even the smallest flicker of a contraction.

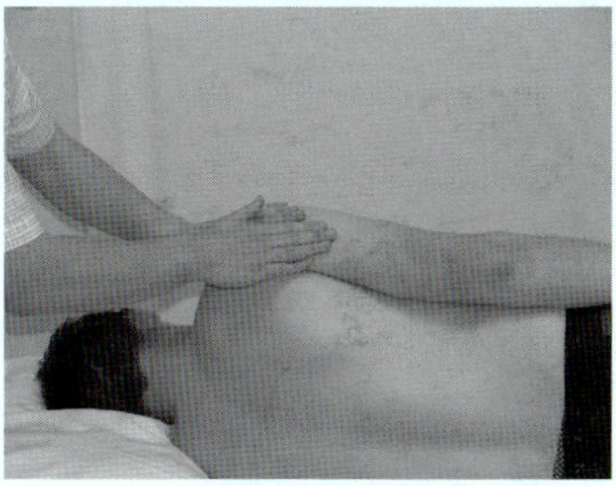

Fig 4.12 Oxford muscle grading for the shoulder extensors – Grades 0 and 1.

Grade 2 – 'Full ROM with the effects of gravity eliminated'

Patient's position: The patient is positioned in side lying on the plinth. Their arm is being supported in full shoulder flexion.

Clinician's position: The clinician is standing by the patient, supporting the limb with one hand under the upper arm and the other supporting just above the wrist.

Command to patient: 'Try and move your arm backwards as far as you can.'

The shoulder has to move through its full range of movement – full flexion to full extension.

Clinical tip: The limb can be heavy, so the safe positioning of the clinician is an essential part of this measurement technique.

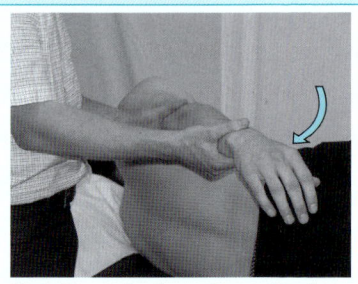

Fig 4.13 Oxford muscle grading for the shoulder extensors – Grade 2. The shoulder has moved from full flexion to full extension (the arm is being moved backwards).

Grade 3 – 'Full ROM against the effects of gravity'

Patient's position: The patient is positioned in standing or sitting, with their arm hanging by their side (neutral). The arm is not starting from full shoulder flexion because gravity would be assisting the movement.

Clinician's position: The clinician is standing behind or to the side of the patient to observe the movement.

Command to patient: 'Lift your arm backwards as far as you can.'

The shoulder has to move from neutral to full extension.

Clinical tip: This application can be performed either sitting or standing; however, for ease of progression to Grades 4 and 5, sitting may be more suitable.

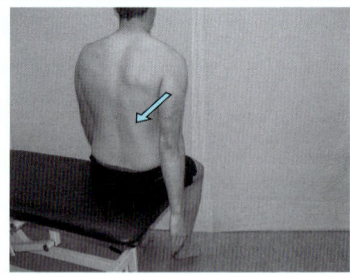

Fig 4.14 Oxford muscle grading for the shoulder extensors – Grade 3. The shoulder is moving from neutral to full extension (the arm is being moved backwards).

Grade 4 – 'Full ROM against minimal resistance'

Patient's position: The patient is positioned in standing or sitting, with their arm hanging by their side (neutral). The arm is not starting from full shoulder flexion because gravity would be assisting the movement.

Clinician's position: The clinician is standing behind the patient, applying a minimal resistance to the distal part of the arm.

Command to patient: 'Lift your arm backwards as far as you can against the minimal resistance.'

The shoulder has to move from neutral to full extension.

Clinical tip: Use the length of lever arm principle to make sure you can apply a consistent resistance to the limb. Ask the patient to start slowly so they can appreciate the amount of resistance. Also, positioning is essential, as the patient needs to be seated so that you can apply even pressure while they approach full range.

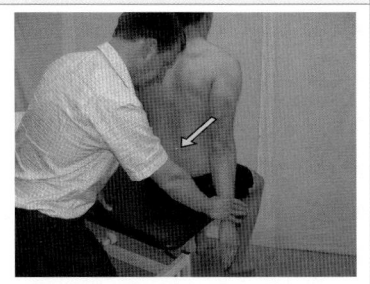

Fig 4.15 Oxford muscle grading for the shoulder extensors – Grades 4 and 5. The shoulder is moving from neutral to full extension (the arm is being moved backwards).

Grade 5 – 'Full ROM against maximal resistance'

Patient's position: The patient is positioned in standing or sitting, with their arm hanging by their side (neutral). The arm is not starting from full shoulder flexion because gravity would be assisting the movement (see Fig. 4.15).

Clinician's position: The clinician is standing behind the patient, applying a maximal resistance to the distal parts of the arm.

Command to patient: 'Lift your arm backwards as far as you can against the maximal resistance.'

The shoulder has to move from neutral to full extension.

Clinical tip: Remember that maximal resistance is related to the patient's maximum and not your maximal. Use the length of lever arm principle to control the resistance through the full range of motion.

Abductors

Grade 0 – 'No contraction' and Grade 1 – 'Flicker of a contraction'

Patient's position: The patient is positioned in supine lying on the plinth, their arm by their side.

Clinician's position: The clinician is standing by the patient, with their hand palpating the middle fibres of deltoid for a contraction.

Command to patient: 'Try and tighten your shoulder muscles and move your arm away from your body.'

Clinical tip: Closely observing and feeling the muscle is essential in enabling the clinician to pick up on even the smallest flicker of a contraction.

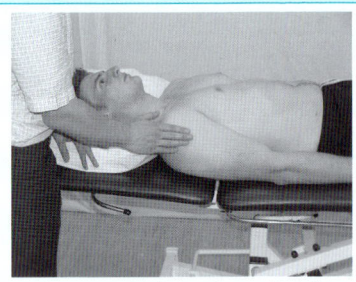

Fig 4.16 Oxford muscle grading for the shoulder abductors – Grades 0 and 1.

Grade 2 – 'Full ROM with the effects of gravity eliminated'

Patient's position: The patient is positioned in supine lying on the plinth. The shoulder is in some degree of flexion to allow the movement to commence in full adduction.

Clinician's position: The clinician is standing by the patient, supporting the limb with one hand under the upper arm and the other supporting just below the elbow.

Command to patient: 'Try and move your arm away from your body, as far as you can.'

The shoulder has to move through its full range of movement – full adduction to full abduction.

Clinical tip: Using a step stance position enables the clinician to take a single step throughout the movement. The limb can be heavy, so the safe positioning of the clinician is an essential part of this measurement technique.

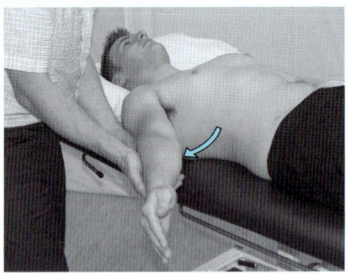

Fig 4.17 Oxford muscle grading for the shoulder abductors – Grade 2. The shoulder is moving from full adduction to full abduction (the arm is being moved out to the side).

Grade 3 – 'Full ROM against the effects of gravity'

Patient's position: The patient is positioned in standing or sitting, with their arm hanging by their side (neutral). The arm is not starting from full shoulder adduction because gravity would be assisting the movement.

Clinician's position: The clinician is positioned to the side of the patient to observe the movement.

Command to patient: 'Lift your arm out and up away from your body as far as you can.'

The shoulder has to move through its full available range of movement – neutral to full abduction.

Clinical tip: Sitting is one of the most suitable and stable positions. From this position it is easy to progress to the testing for Grades 4 and 5.

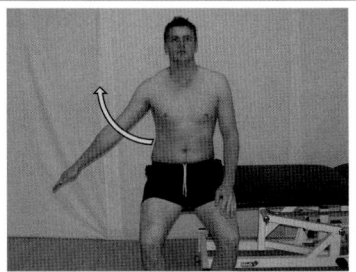

Fig 4.18 Oxford muscle grading for the shoulder abductors – Grade 3. The shoulder is moving from neutral to full abduction (the arm is being raised towards the ceiling).

Grade 4 – 'Full ROM against minimal resistance'

Patient's position: The patient is positioned in standing or sitting, with their arm hanging by their side (neutral). The arm is not starting from full shoulder adduction because gravity would be assisting the movement.

Clinician's position: The clinician is standing to the side of the patient, applying a minimal resistance to the distal part of the arm.

Command to patient: 'Lift your arm out sideways as far as you can against the maximal resistance.'

The shoulder has to move through its full available range of movement – neutral to full abduction.

Clinical tip: Use the length of lever arm principle to make sure you can apply a consistent resistance to the limb. Ask the patient to start slowly so they can appreciate the amount of resistance. Also, positioning is essential, as the patient needs to be seated so that you can apply even pressure while they approach full range.

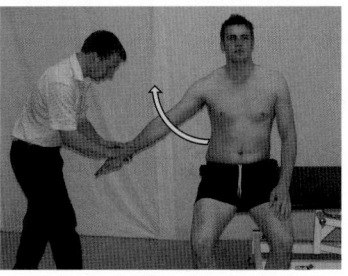

Fig 4.19 Oxford muscle grading for the shoulder abductors – Grades 4 and 5. The shoulder is moving from neutral to full abduction (the arm is being raised towards the ceiling).

Grade 5 – 'Full ROM against maximal resistance'

Patient's position: The patient is positioned in standing or sitting, with their arm hanging by their side (neutral). The arm is not starting from full shoulder adduction because gravity would be assisting the movement (see Fig. 4.19).

Clinician's position: The clinician is standing to the side of the patient, applying a maximal resistance to the distal part of the arm.

Command to patient: 'Lift your arm out sideways as far as you can against the maximal resistance.'

The shoulder has to move through its full available range of movement – neutral to full abduction.

Clinical tip: Remember that maximal resistance is related to the patient's maximum and not your maximal. Use the length of lever arm principle to control the resistance through the full range of motion.

Adductors

Grade 0 – 'No contraction' and Grade 1 – 'Flicker of a contraction'

Patient's position: The patient is positioned in supine lying on the plinth, with the arm to be tested positioned slightly away from the body.

Clinician's position: The clinician is standing by the patient with their hand palpating pectoralis major for signs of a contraction.

Command to patient: 'Try and tighten your shoulder muscles and move your arm towards your body.'

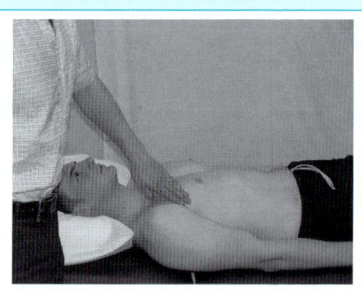

Fig 4.20 Oxford muscle grading for the shoulder adductors – Grades 0 and 1.

Clinical tip: Obviously the trunk is in the way of a possible true adduction movement; therefore, the clinician is reminded that adaptations to this procedure may be necessary.

Pectoralis major can be felt in the upper part of the chest from both its clavicular and sternocostal attachments.

Measurement

Grade 2 – 'Full ROM with the effects of gravity eliminated'

Patient's position: The patient is positioned in supine lying on the plinth, their shoulder in some degree of flexion and their arm in full abduction.

Clinician's position: The clinician is standing by the patient, supporting the limb, with one hand under the upper arm and the other supporting just below the elbow.

Command to patient: 'Try and move your arm across your body as far as you can.'

The shoulder has to move through its full range of movement – from full abduction to full adduction.

Clinical tip: Again, the trunk will interfere with the application of the true movement of adduction, therefore the shoulder has to be in 20–30° of flexion to allow the arm to move across the body into adduction.

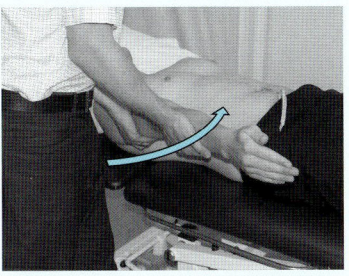

Fig 4.21 Oxford muscle grading for the shoulder adductors – Grade 2. The shoulder is moving from full abduction to full adduction (the arm is moved across the abdomen).

Grade 3 – 'Full ROM against the effects of gravity'

Patient's position: The patient is positioned in standing, with their arm hanging free by their side (neutral). The arm is not starting from full shoulder abduction because gravity would be assisting the movement.

Clinician's position: The clinician is positioned in front or to the side of the patient to enable them to observe the movement.

Command to patient: 'Lift your arm across your body as far as you can.'

The shoulder has moved through its full available range of movement – from neutral to full adduction.

Clinical tip: Again, the trunk will interfere with the application of the true movement of adduction, therefore the shoulder has to be in 20–30° of flexion to allow the arm to move across the body into adduction.

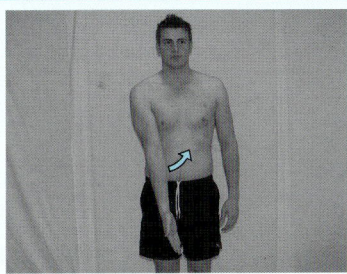

Fig 4.22 Oxford muscle grading for the shoulder adductors – Grade 3. The shoulder has to move from neutral to full adduction (across the body).

THE SHOULDER JOINT

Grade 4 – 'Full ROM against minimal resistance'

Patient's position: The patient is positioned in standing, with their arm hanging free by their side (neutral). The arm is not starting from full shoulder abduction because gravity would be assisting the movement.

Clinician's position: The clinician is standing to the side of the patient, applying a minimal resistance to the distal part of the arm.

Command to patient: 'Move your arm across your body as far as you can against the minimal resistance.'

The shoulder has moved through its full available range of movement – from neutral to full adduction. The trunk will interfere with the application of the true movement of adduction, therefore the shoulder has to be in 20–30° of flexion to allow the arm to move across the body into adduction.

Clinical tip: Use the length of lever arm principle to make sure you can apply a consistent resistance to the limb. Ask the patient to start slowly so they can appreciate the amount of resistance. Also, positioning is essential, as the patient needs to be seated so that you can apply even pressure while they approach full range.

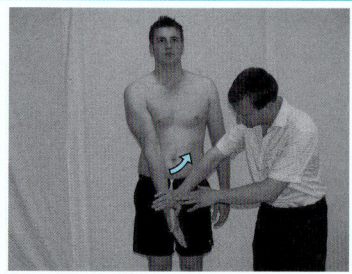

Fig 4.23 Oxford muscle grading for the shoulder adductors – Grades 4 and 5. The shoulder has moved from neutral to full adduction (across the body).

Grade 5 – 'Full ROM against maximal resistance'

Patient's position: The patient is positioned in standing, with their arm hanging free by their side (neutral). The arm is not starting from full shoulder abduction because gravity would be assisting the movement (see Fig. 4.23).

Clinician's position: The clinician is standing to the side of the patient, applying the maximal resistance to the distal part of the arm.

Command to patient: 'Move your arm across your body as far as you can against the maximal resistance.'

The shoulder has moved through its full available range of movement – from neutral to full adduction. The trunk will interfere with the application of the true movement of adduction, therefore the shoulder has to be in 20–30° of flexion to allow the arm to move across the body into adduction.

Clinical tip: Remember that maximal resistance is related to the patient's maximum and not your maximal. Use the length of lever arm principle to control the resistance through full range of motion.

Measurement

Medial (internal) rotators

Grade 0 – 'No contraction' and Grade 1 – 'Flicker of a contraction'

Patient's position: The patient is positioned in supine lying, with the palm of the arm to be tested resting on the patient's abdomen.

Clinician's position: The clinician is standing by the patient, with their hand palpating pectoralis major for a sign of a contraction.

Command to patient: 'Try and push your palm into your abdomen.'

Clinical tip: Closely observing and feeling the tendon is essential in enabling the clinician to pick up on even the smallest flicker of a contraction.

Pectoralis major can be felt in the upper part of the chest from both its clavicular and sternocostal attachments.

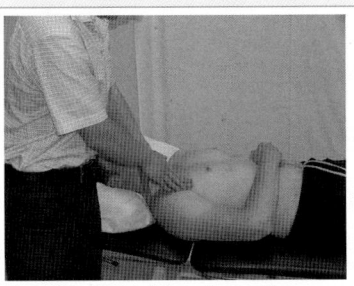

Fig 4.24 Oxford muscle grading for the shoulder medial (internal) rotators – Grades 0 and 1.

Grade 2 – 'Full ROM with the effects of gravity eliminated'

Patient's position: The patient is positioned in sitting or in long sitting on the plinth, with the shoulder in neutral, the elbow in 90° of flexion and in mid-supination/pronation.

Clinician's position: The clinician is standing by the patient, with one hand under the olecranon of the elbow supporting the weight of the limb and the other supporting proximal to the wrist.

Command to patient: 'Try to move your hand towards your body as far as you can, keeping your upper arm by your side.'

The shoulder has to move through its full range of movement – full lateral rotation to full medial rotation.

Clinical tip: The trunk will interfere with the application of the true movement of medial rotation, therefore adaptation may be required. The limb can be heavy, so the safe positioning of the clinician is an essential part of this measurement technique.

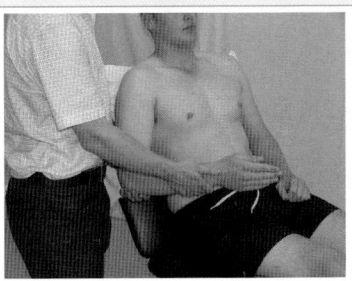

Fig 4.25 Oxford muscle grading for the shoulder medial (internal) rotators – Grade 2. The shoulder is moving from full lateral rotation to full medial rotation (the forearm and hand are moving in towards the abdomen).

THE SHOULDER JOINT

Grade 3 – 'Full ROM against the effects of gravity'

Patient's position: The patient is positioned in supine lying or 45° right side lying on the plinth, their shoulder in lateral rotation, elbow in 90° of flexion and the forearm in the mid-position.

Clinician's position: The clinician is standing by the side of the patient to observe the movement.

Command to patient: 'Move your arm inwards until your palm reaches your abdomen, or as far as you can.'

The shoulder has to move through its full range of movement – full lateral rotation to full medial rotation.

Clinical tip: The trunk may interfere with the full range of medial rotation.

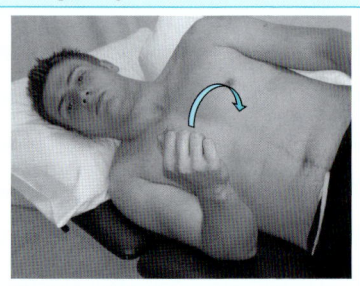

Fig 4.26 Oxford muscle grading for the shoulder medial (internal) rotators – Grade 3. The shoulder is moving from full lateral rotation to full medial rotation (the forearm and hand are moving in towards the abdomen).

Grade 4 – 'Full ROM against minimal resistance'

Patient's position: The patient is positioned in supine lying or 45° right side lying on the plinth, their shoulder in lateral rotation, elbow in 90° of flexion and the forearm in the mid-position.

Clinician's position: The clinician is standing by the side of the patient, applying a minimal resistance to the distal medial area of the wrist, simultaneously supporting the arm at the elbow.

Command to patient: 'Try and move your arm so that your palm reaches your abdomen, against the minimal resistance.'

The shoulder has to move through its full range of movement – full lateral rotation to full medial rotation.

Clinical tip: The elbow is in 90° of flexion, which means that the clinician can use the length of lever arm principle and induce a mechanical advantage over the patient.

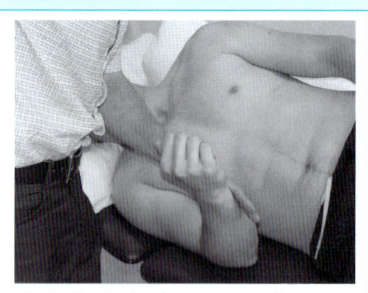

Fig 4.27 Oxford muscle grading for the shoulder medial (internal) rotators – Grades 4 and 5. The shoulder is moving from full lateral rotation to full medial rotation (the forearm and hand are moving in towards the abdomen).

Grade 5 – 'Full ROM against maximal resistance'

Patient's position: The patient is positioned in supine lying or 45° right side lying on the plinth, their shoulder in lateral rotation, elbow in 90° of flexion and the forearm in the mid-position (see Fig. 4.27).

Clinician's position: The clinician is standing by the side of the patient, applying a maximal resistance to the distal area of the wrist, simultaneously supporting the arm at the elbow.

Command to patient: 'Try and move your arm so that your palm reaches your abdomen, against the maximal resistance.'

The shoulder has to move through its full range of movement – full lateral rotation to full medial rotation.

Clinical tip: The elbow is in 90° of flexion, which means that the clinician can use the length of lever arm principle and induce a mechanical advantage over the patient.

Remember that maximal resistance is related to the patient's maximum and not your maximal.

Grade 4 – 'Full ROM against minimal resistance' – alternative

Patient's position: The patient is positioned in standing or sitting, with their shoulder in lateral rotation, elbow in 90° of flexion and the forearm in the mid-position.

Clinician's position: The clinician is standing by the side of the patient, applying a minimal resistance to the distal lateral area of the wrist, simultaneously supporting the arm at the elbow.

Command to patient: 'Try and move your arm so that your palm moves in towards your abdomen as far as you can, against the minimal resistance.'

The shoulder has to move through its full range of movement – full lateral rotation to full medial rotation.

Clinical tip: Remember that the clinician will have a large mechanical advantage in this position; therefore, consideration should be given to the amount of resistance required during this technique.

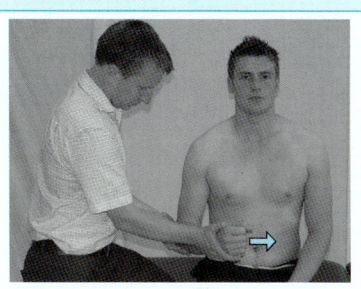

Fig 4.28 Oxford muscle grading for the shoulder medial (internal) rotators – Grades 4 and 5. The shoulder is moving from full lateral rotation to full medial rotation (the forearm and hand are moving in towards the abdomen).

THE SHOULDER JOINT

> ### Grade 5 – 'Full ROM against maximal resistance' – alternative
>
> **Patient's position:** The patient is positioned in standing or sitting, with their shoulder in lateral (external) rotation, the elbow in 90° of flexion and the forearm in the mid-position (see Fig. 4.28).
>
> **Clinician's position:** The clinician is standing by the side of the patient, applying a maximal resistance to the distal lateral area of the wrist, simultaneously supporting the arm at the elbow.
>
> **Command to patient:** 'Try and move your arm so that your palm reaches your abdomen, against the maximal resistance.'
>
> The shoulder has to move through its full range of movement – full lateral rotation to full medial rotation.
>
> **Clinical tip:** The elbow is in 90° of flexion, which means that the clinician can use the length of lever principle and induce a mechanical advantage over the patient.
>
> Remember that maximal resistance is related to the patient's maximum and not your maximal.

> ### Lateral (external) rotators
>
> ### Grade 0 – 'No contraction' and Grade 1 – 'Flicker of a contraction'
>
> **Patient's position:** The patient is positioned in supine lying on the plinth, with the palm of the arm to be tested resting on the patient's abdomen; or sitting, with their arm supported on pillows. Their shoulder is in medial rotation, the elbow is in 90° of flexion and the forearm is in the mid-position.
>
> **Clinician's position:** The clinician is standing by the patient, with their hand palpating the lateral border of the scapula for teres minor.
>
> **Fig 4.29** Oxford muscle grading for the shoulder lateral (external) rotators – Grades 0 and 1.
>
> **Command to patient:** 'Try and move your arm out or try and lift your hand away from your abdomen.'
>
> **Clinical tip:** Closely observing and feeling the muscle is essential in enabling the clinician to pick up on even the smallest flicker of a contraction.
>
> Teres minor may be felt mid-way up the lateral border of the scapula.

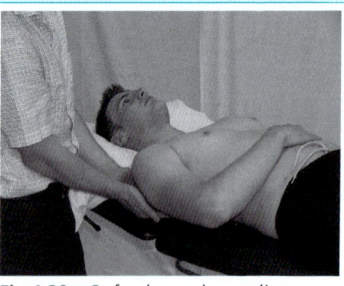

Measurement

Grade 2 – 'Full ROM with the effects of gravity eliminated'

Patient's position: The patient is positioned in sitting or long sitting on the plinth, with their shoulder in medial rotation, their elbow in 90° of flexion and in the mid-supination/pronation position.

Clinician's position: The clinician is positioned by the patient, with one hand under the olecranon of the elbow, supporting the weight of the limb, and the other supporting proximal to the wrist.

Command to patient: 'Try to move your hand away from your body as far as you can, keeping your upper arm by your side.'

The shoulder has to move through its full range of movement – full medial rotation to full lateral rotation.

Clinical tip: It is important for the clinician to support the arm, but not assist in the movement as this negates the principle of the patient performing the movement.

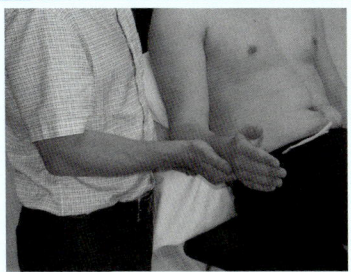

Fig 4.30 Oxford muscle grading for the shoulder lateral (external) rotators – Grade 2. The shoulder is moving from full medial rotation to full lateral rotation (the forearm and hand are moving away from the abdomen).

Grade 3 – 'Full ROM against the effects of gravity'

Patient's position: The patient is positioned in side lying on the plinth, with their shoulder in medial (internal) rotation, their elbow in 90° of flexion and the forearm in the mid-position, with their hand on their abdomen.

Clinician's position: The clinician is standing by the patient, in a suitable position to observe the movement.

Command to patient: 'Take your palm away from your abdomen as far as you can, keeping your upper arm against the side of your body.'

The shoulder has to move through its full range of movement – full medial rotation to full lateral rotation.

Clinical tip: The patient may need supporting in this position either by the clinician or by pillows on the plinth.

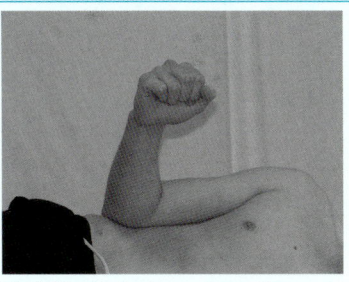

Fig 4.31 Oxford muscle grading for the shoulder lateral (external) rotators – Grade 3. The shoulder is moving from full medial rotation to full lateral rotation (the forearm and hand are moving up towards the ceiling).

THE SHOULDER JOINT

Grade 4 – 'Full ROM against minimal resistance'

Patient's position: The patient is positioned in standing or sitting, with their shoulder in medial rotation, their elbow in 90° of flexion and the forearm in the mid-position.

Clinician's position: The clinician is standing by the side of the patient, applying a minimal resistance to the distal lateral area of the wrist, simultaneously supporting the arm at the elbow.

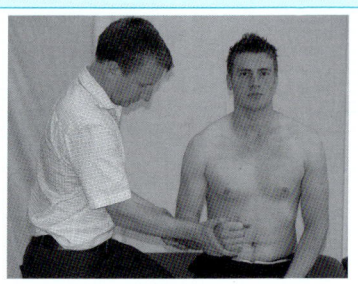

Fig 4.32 Oxford muscle grading for the shoulder lateral (external) rotators – Grades 4 and 5. The shoulder is moving from full medial rotation to full lateral rotation (the forearm and hand are moving away from the abdomen).

Command to patient: 'Try and move your arm so that your palm moves away from your abdomen as far as you can, against the minimal resistance.'

The shoulder has to move through its full range of movement – full medial rotation to full lateral rotation.

Clinical tip: Remember that the clinician will have a large mechanical advantage in this position; therefore consideration should be given to the amount of resistance required during this technique.

Grade 5 – 'Full ROM against maximal resistance'

Patient's position: The patient is positioned in standing or sitting, with their shoulder in medial (internal) rotation, their elbow in 90° of flexion and the forearm in the mid-position (see Fig. 4.32).

Clinician's position: The clinician is standing by the side of the patient, applying a maximal resistance to the distal lateral area of the wrist, simultaneously supporting the arm at the elbow.

Command to patient: 'Try and move your arm so that your palm moves away from your abdomen as far as you can, against the maximal resistance.'

The shoulder has to move through its full range of movement – full medial rotation to full lateral rotation.

Clinical tip: The elbow is in 90° of flexion, which means that the clinician can use the length of lever principle and induce a mechanical advantage over the patient.

Remember that maximal resistance is related to the patient's maximum and not your maximal.

Measurement 123

Notes

Treatment record

THE SHOULDER JOINT

Notes

Treatment record

CHAPTER 5

The elbow joint

ANATOMY   125
  The elbow joint   125
  The superior radioulnar joint   125
  The inferior radioulnar joint   126
Bony landmarks to be palpated   126
Ligaments   126
Muscles   127
  Flexors   127
  Extensors   128
  Supinators   129
  Pronators   130
MEASUREMENT   131

Range of movement   131
  Flexion   131
  Extension   132
  Supination   133
  Pronation   134
  Observational/reflective checklist   136
Joint girth   137
  Elbow   137
Muscle strength: Oxford muscle grading   139
  Extensors   139
  Flexors   141
  Supinators   144
  Pronators   146

ANATOMY

The elbow joint
1. The elbow joint is a synovial hinge joint.
2. The trochlear surface of the humerus articulates with the trochlear notch of the ulna and the capitulum of the humerus articulates with the head of the radius.
3. A fibrous capsule completely encloses the elbow joint, including the superior radioulnar joint.
4. The elbow joint has strong collateral ligaments – the radial and ulnar collateral ligaments.
5. The movements that take place at the elbow joint are flexion and extension.

The superior radioulnar joint
1. This is a synovial pivot joint.

2. It is an articulation between the head of the radius, rotating within the fibro-osseous ring formed by the radial notch of the ulna and the annular ligament.
3. The movements that take place are pronation and supination.

The inferior radioulnar joint
1. This is a synovial pivot joint.
2. It is an articulation between the head of the ulna and the ulnar notch on the lower end of the radius.
3. The joint is closed inferiorly by an articular disc, which passes between the radius and the ulna.
4. The movements that take place are pronation and supination.

BONY LANDMARKS TO BE PALPATED

The humerus – medial epicondyle, medial supracondylar ridge, lateral epicondyle and lateral supracondylar ridge.
The radius – the head.
The ulna – the olecranon process.

LIGAMENTS

Table 5.1

The ligaments

Articulation	Ligament	Origin	Insertion	Limitation to movement
Elbow joint	Ulnar collateral	Medial epicondyle of the humerus	Medial edge of the coronoid process of the ulna	Valgus stress of the elbow
Elbow joint	Radial collateral	Lateral epicondyle of the humerus	Common extensor origin and the annular ligament of the radius	Varus stress of the elbow
Superior radioulnar joint	Annular	Anterior aspect of the radial notch of the ulna	Posterior aspect of the radial notch of the ulna, encasing the head of radius	Restraining ligament of the head of radius
Superior radioulnar joint	Quadrate	Radial notch of the ulna	Medial surface of the neck of the radius	To maintain tension between the radius and ulna in supination and pronation

MUSCLES
Flexors

Table 5.2

The flexors of the elbow				
Muscle	Origin	Insertion	Nerve supply	Action(s)
Biceps brachii	Long head = superior glenoid tubercle of scapula Short head = coracoid process of the scapula	Bicipital aponeurosis and the radial tuberosity	Musculocutaneous nerve C5, 6	Long head = flexion of the shoulder joint Long head and short head = flexion and supination of the elbow
Brachialis	Distal two-thirds of the anterior aspect of the shaft of the humerus	Brachialis impression on inferior part of coronoid process and tuberosity of ulna	Musculocutaneous nerve C5,6	Flexion of the elbow
Brachioradialis	Upper two-thirds of the lateral supracondylar ridge of the humerus and the lateral intermuscular septum	Lateral surface of the radius above the styloid process	Radial nerve C5, 6	Flexion of the elbow, and it pulls the elbow into the mid-position from either the supinated or pronated position
Pronator teres	Medial supracondylar ridge, intermuscular septum, and medial epicondyle of humerus, pronator ridge of the ulna	Roughened area on the lateral surface of the radius	Median nerve C6, 7	Pronation of the forearm and flexion of the elbow

Extensors

Table 5.3

The extensors of the elbow				
Muscle	Origin	Insertion	Nerve supply	Action(s)
Triceps brachii	Lateral head = above the spiral groove on the posterior surface of the humerus Long head = infraglenoid tubercle of the scapula Medial head = below the spiral groove on the medial aspect of the posterior surface of the humerus	Posterior part of the olecranon of the ulna	Radial nerve C6, 7, 8	Extension of the shoulder from a flexed position, adduction of the shoulder joint and extension of the elbow
Anconeus	Posterior surface of the lateral epicondyle of the humerus	Lateral surface of the olecranon of the ulna	Radial nerve C7, 8	Elbow extension

Supinators

Table 5.4

The supinators of the forearm				
Muscle	Origin	Insertion	Nerve supply	Action(s)
Supinator	Inferior aspect of the lateral epicondyle of the humerus, radial collateral ligament	Posterior, anterior and lateral aspects of the radius	Posterior interosseous branch of the radial nerve C5, 6	Supination of the forearm
Biceps brachii	Long head = superior glenoid tubercle of the scapula Short head = coracoid process of the scapula	Bicipital aponeurosis and the radial tuberosity	Musculocutaneous nerve C5, 6	Long head = flexion of the shoulder joint Long head and short head = flexion and supination of the elbow
Brachioradialis	Upper two-thirds of the lateral supracondylar ridge of the humerus and the lateral intermuscular septum	Lateral surface of the radius above the styloid process	Radial nerve C5, 6	Flexion of the elbow, and it pulls the elbow into the mid-position from either the supinated or pronated position

Pronators

Table 5.5

The pronators of the forearm

Muscle	Origin	Insertion	Nerve supply	Action(s)
Pronator teres	Medial supracondylar ridge, intermuscular septum, and medial epicondyle of humerus, pronator ridge of the ulna	Roughened area on the lateral surface of the radius	Median nerve C6, 7	Pronation of the forearm and flexion of the elbow
Pronator quadratus	Lower quarter of the anterior surface of the ulna	Lower quarter of the anterior surface of the radius	Anterior interosseous branch of the median nerve C8, T1	Pronation of the forearm
Brachioradialis	Upper two-thirds of the lateral supracondylar ridge of the humerus and the lateral intermuscular septum	Lateral surface of the radius above the styloid process	Radial nerve C5, 6	Flexion of the elbow, and it pulls the elbow into the mid-position from either the supinated or pronated position

MEASUREMENT

RANGE OF MOVEMENT
Flexion

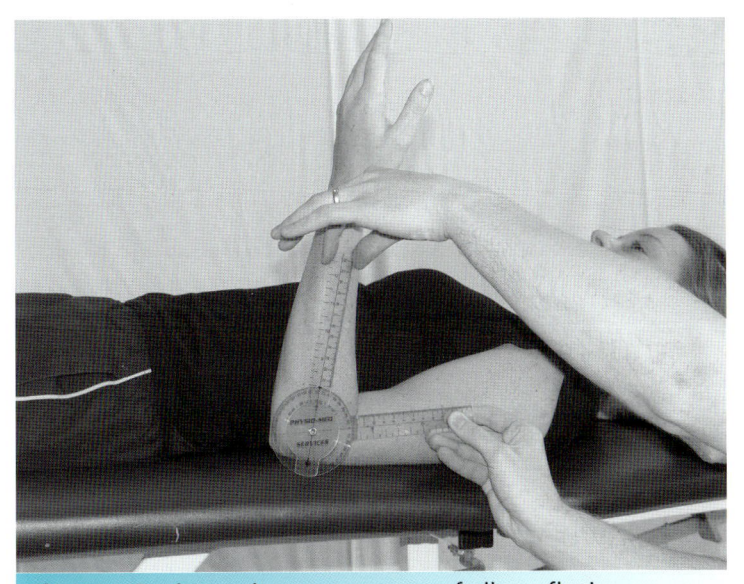

Fig 5.1 Goniometric measurement of elbow flexion.

Starting position: The patient is positioned in supine lying on the plinth. Their arm is in the anatomical position, with the elbow in 0° of extension.
Stabilization: The clinician stabilizes the humerus.
Goniometer axis: The axis of the goniometer is placed over the lateral epicondyle of the humerus.
Stationary arm: This is parallel to the longitudinal axis of the humerus, pointing towards the tip of the acromion process.
Moveable arm: This is parallel to the longitudinal axis of the radius, pointing towards the styloid process of the radius.
End position: The forearm is moved in an anterior direction so the hand approximates to the shoulder.

NB: It may be necessary to reposition the stationary and moveable arms of the goniometer prior to taking the reading, as they may have moved when the patient flexed their elbow.

Extension

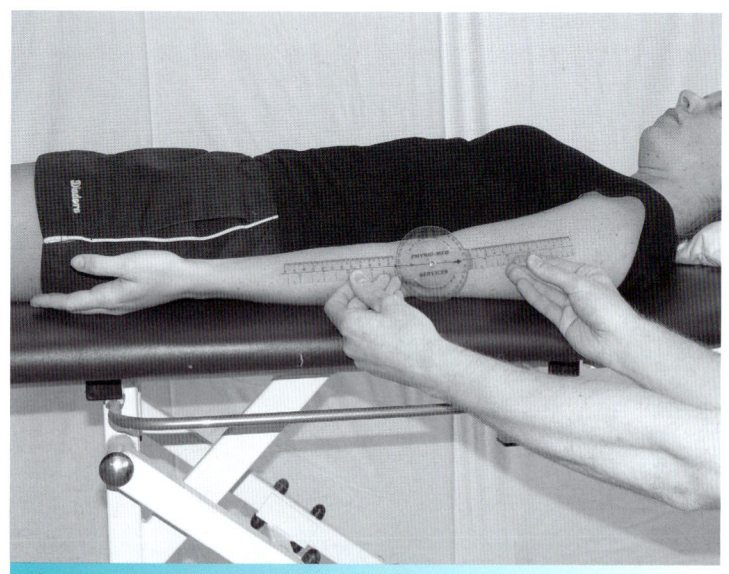

Fig 5.2 Goniometric measurement of elbow extension.

Starting position: The patient is positioned in supine lying on the plinth. Their arm is in the anatomical position, with the elbow in 0° of extension.
Stabilization: The clinician stabilizes the humerus.
Goniometer axis: The axis of the goniometer is placed over the lateral epicondyle of the humerus.
Stationary arm: This is parallel to the longitudinal axis of the humerus, pointing towards the tip of the acromion process.
Moveable arm: This is parallel to the longitudinal axis of the radius, pointing towards the styloid process of the radius.
End position: The clinician encourages the patient to straighten their elbow as much as possible.

Supination

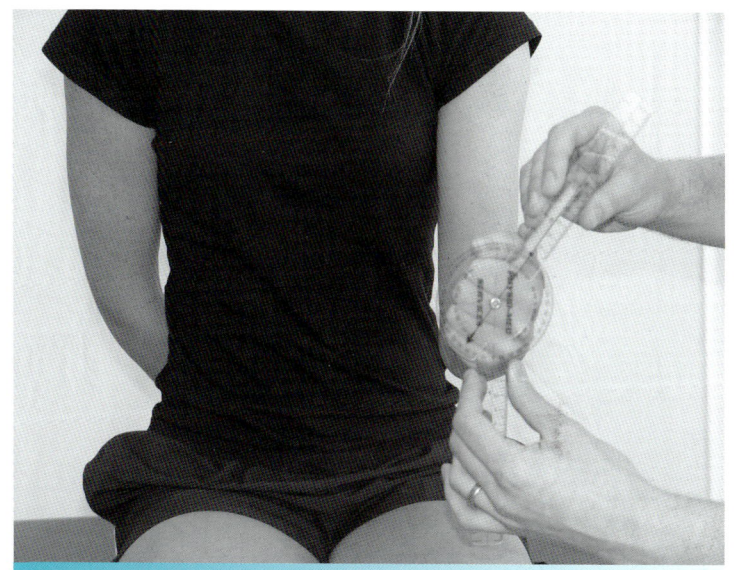

Fig 5.3 Goniometric measurement of elbow supination.

Starting position: The patient is sitting, their shoulder is adducted, with the elbow flexed to 90°, the forearm in the mid-position and the wrist in neutral. A pencil is held in the tightly closed fist, with the pencil protruding from the radial (thumb) aspect of the hand.
Stabilization: The clinician stabilizes the humerus.
Goniometer axis: The axis of the goniometer is placed over the middle of the shaft of the third metacarpal.
Stationary arm: This is perpendicular to the floor.
Moveable arm: This is parallel to the pencil.
End position: The patient is asked to rotate their forearm laterally (externally) from the mid-position so the palm is facing upwards (supination).
Trick movements: Altered grip/wrist grip, shoulder movements.

> **Clinical tip**
> Ensure the arm remains adducted while performing the movement.

THE ELBOW JOINT

Pronation

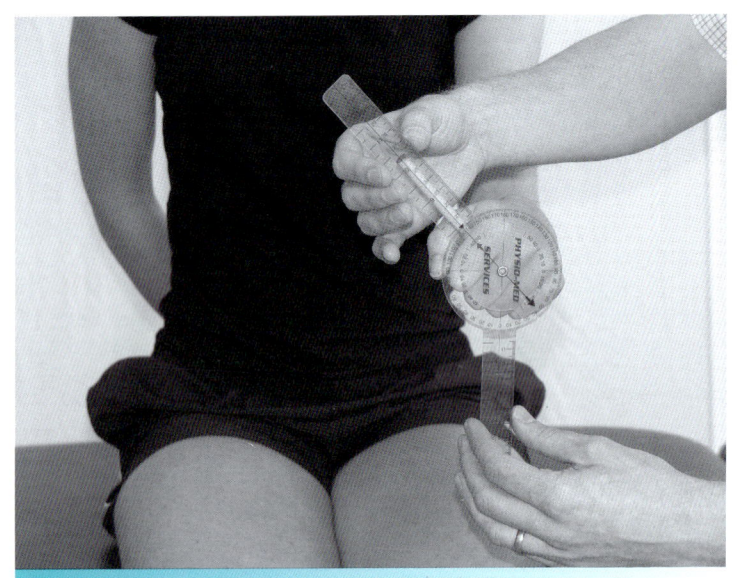

Fig 5.4 Goniometric measurement of elbow pronation.

Starting position: The patient is sitting, their shoulder is adducted, with the elbow flexed to 90°, the forearm in the mid-position and the wrist in neutral. A pencil is held in the tightly closed fist, with the pencil protruding from the radial (thumb) aspect of the hand.
Stabilization: The clinician stabilizes the humerus.
Goniometer axis: The axis of the goniometer is placed over the middle of the shaft of the third metacarpal.
Stationary arm: This is perpendicular to the floor.
Moveable arm: This is parallel to the pencil.
End position: The patient is asked to rotate their forearm medially (internally), from the mid-position, so the palm is facing downwards (pronation).
Trick movements: Altered grip/wrist grip, shoulder movements.

> **Clinical tip**
> Ensure the arm remains adducted while performing the movement.

Measurement   135

Notes

Treatment record

THE ELBOW JOINT

Observational/reflective checklist

Observational/reflective checklist			
Observation		Y/N	Comments
Introduction and preparation for the skill	Was the treatment area properly prepared for the patient, e.g. pillow, blanket, safe environment, etc.?		
	Did the therapist introduce him/herself?		
	Was the patient comfortable?		
	Was the patient adequately exposed/draped?		
	Was an explanation of the procedure given?		
	Was the explanation clear and succinct?		
	Was consent obtained?		
Performing the skill	Was the plinth set at the correct height?		
	Was the therapist's posture compromised?		
	Did the therapist identify the joint and other relevant bony landmarks?		
	Was the goniometer correctly aligned?		
	Was the reading of the joint range of movement accurate?		
	Did the therapist compare both sides of the body?		
Safe and effective performance of the technique	Was the procedure carried out with due care and attention?		
How would you rate the proficiency in the overall performance of the skill?	Excellent		
	Very good		
	Good		
	Satisfactory		
	Borderline		
	Fail		

Measurement

JOINT GIRTH
Elbow

The elbow joint can be identified by drawing a line 1 cm below the lateral epicondyle of the humerus and 2 cm below the medial epicondyle of the humerus. It can also be felt posteriorly, between the head of the radius and the capitulum of the humerus.

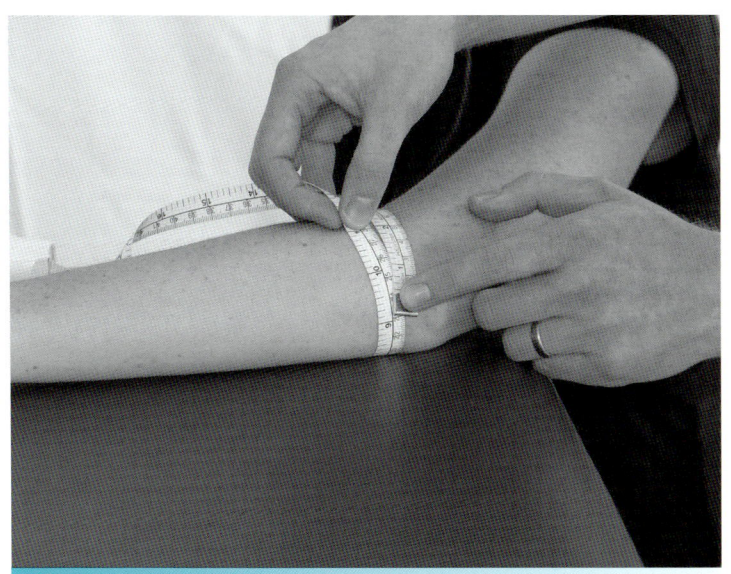

Fig 5.5 Measurement of the girth of the elbow joint.

Patient's position: The patient is positioned in sitting, their arm supported on a table or plinth. The elbow joint is encircled with a tape measure at the joint line. The circumferential measurements are then recorded.

Repeat the procedure on the other elbow joint.

Repeat the procedure three times and produce an average score.

> Points to note:
>   The state of the tape measure – is it stretched?
>   The muscles must be relaxed.
>   Keep the tape measure straight (not twisted).
>   Measure consistently – at the top/bottom of the tape, and either in centimetres or in inches.

138 THE ELBOW JOINT

Notes

Treatment record

Measurement

MUSCLE STRENGTH: OXFORD MUSCLE GRADING

Extensors

Grade 0 – 'No contraction' and Grade 1 – 'Flicker of a contraction'

Patient's position: The patient is positioned in sitting, their arm supported on a table or plinth and their shoulder in 90° of abduction.

Clinician's position: The clinician is positioned by the side of the patient, palpating the triceps area of the upper arm.

Command to patient: 'Try and make the muscles on this part of your arm tighten/try and straighten your elbow.'

Clinical tip: Closely observing and feeling the muscle is essential in enabling the clinician to pick up on even the smallest flicker of a contraction.

The triceps muscle can be felt on the posterior aspect of the arm.

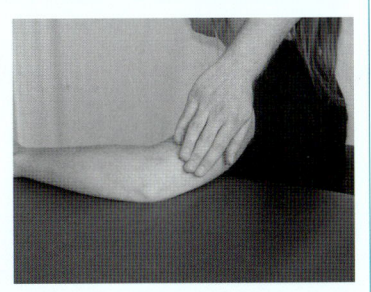

Fig 5.6 Oxford muscle grading for the elbow extensors – Grades 0 and 1.

Grade 2 – 'Full ROM with the effects of gravity eliminated'

Patient's position: The patient is positioned in sitting, their arm supported on a table or plinth; their shoulder is in 90° of abduction and their elbow in full flexion.

Clinician's position: The clinician is standing by the patient, supporting the weight of the arm, both proximally and distally.

Command to patient: 'Try and straighten your elbow as far as you can.'

The elbow has to move through its full range of movement – full flexion to full extension.

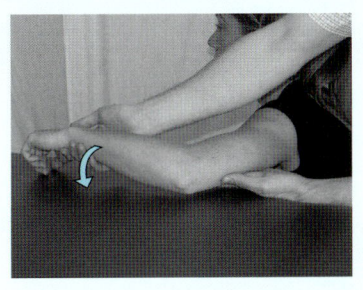

Fig 5.7 Oxford muscle grading for the elbow extensors – Grade 2. The elbow is moving from full flexion to full extension (the elbow is straightening).

Grade 3 – 'Full ROM against the effects of gravity'

Patient's position: The patient is positioned in sitting, with their shoulder in extension and their elbow in as much flexion as they can obtain.

Clinician's position: The clinician is standing by the patient, stabilizing the upper arm and observing the movement.

Command to patient: 'Try and straighten your elbow as far as you can.'

The elbow has to move through its full range of movement – full flexion to full extension.

Clinical tip: Initially, the movement is assisted by gravity.

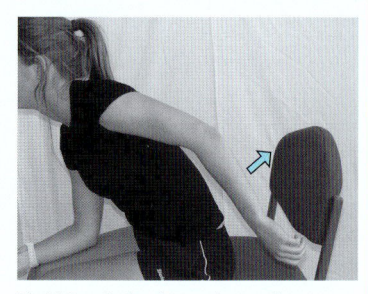

Fig 5.8 Oxford muscle grading for the elbow extensors – Grade 3. The elbow is moving from full flexion to full extension (the elbow is straightening).

Grade 4 – 'Full ROM against minimal resistance'

Patient's position: The patient is positioned in sitting, with their arm supported on a table or plinth; their shoulder is in 90° of flexion, with the elbow in full flexion and the forearm supinated.

Clinician's position: The clinician is standing by the patient, applying a minimal resistance to the distal forearm as the subject extends their elbow.

Command to patient: 'Try and straighten your elbow as far as you can against the minimal resistance.'

The elbow has to move through its full range of movement – full flexion to full extension.

Clinical tip: Use the length of lever arm principle to make sure you can apply a consistent resistance to the limb. Ask the patient to start slowly so they can appreciate the amount of resistance.

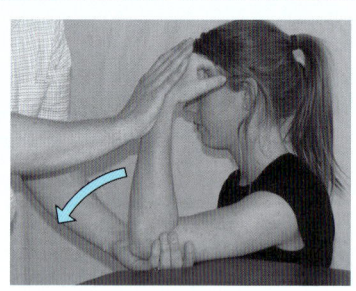

Fig 5.9 Oxford muscle grading for the elbow extensors – Grades 4 and 5. The elbow is moving from full flexion to full extension (the elbow is straightening).

Measurement

Grade 5 – 'Full ROM against maximal resistance'

Patient's position: The patient is positioned in sitting, with their arm supported on a table or plinth; their shoulder is in 90° of flexion, the elbow in full flexion and the forearm supinated (see Fig. 5.9).

Clinician's position: The clinician is standing by the patient, applying a maximal resistance to the distal forearm as the subject extends their elbow.

Command to patient: 'Try and straighten your elbow as far as you can against the maximal resistance.'

The elbow has to move through its full range of movement – full flexion to full extension.

Clinical tip: Use the length of lever arm principle to make sure you can apply a consistent resistance to the limb. Ask the patient to start slowly so they can appreciate the amount of resistance.

Flexors

Grade 0 – 'No contraction' and Grade 1 – 'Flicker of a contraction'

Patient's position: The patient is positioned in sitting, with their arm supported on a table or plinth; their shoulder is in 90° of flexion and their elbow is fully extended.

Clinician's position: The clinician is standing by the patient, palpating the biceps brachii region of their upper arm.

Command to patient: 'Try and make the muscles on this part of your arm tighten/try and move your hand towards your shoulder.'

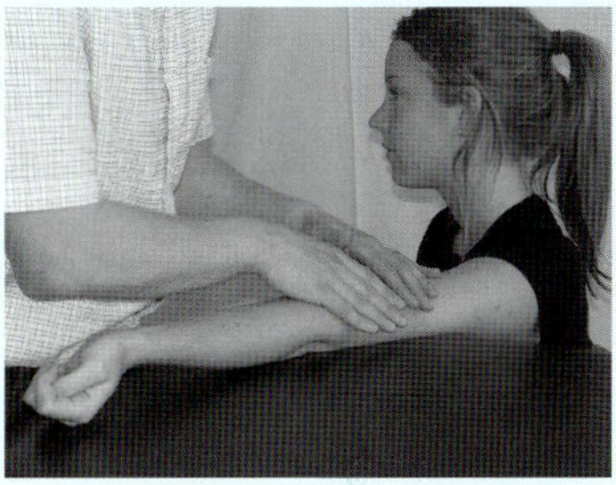

Fig 5.10 Oxford muscle grading for the elbow flexors – Grades 0 and 1.

Clinical tip: Closely observing and feeling the muscle is essential in enabling the clinician to pick up on even the smallest flicker of a contraction.

142 THE ELBOW JOINT

Grade 2 – 'Full ROM with the effects of gravity eliminated'

Patient's position: The patient is positioned in sitting, with their arm supported on a table or plinth; their shoulder is in 90° of abduction and their elbow is fully extended.

Clinician's position: The clinician is standing by the patient, supporting the weight of their upper arm and forearm.

Command to patient: 'Try and take your hand up to your shoulder as far as you can.'

The elbow has to move through its full range of movement – full extension to full flexion.

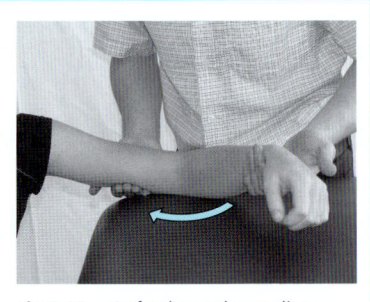

Fig 5.11 Oxford muscle grading for the elbow flexors – Grade 2. The elbow is moving from full extension to full flexion (the hand is moving up towards the shoulder).

Grade 3 – 'Full ROM against the effects of gravity'

Patient's position: The patient is positioned in sitting, with their arm supported on a table or plinth; their shoulder is in 90° of abduction, elbow fully extended and their forearm supinated.

Clinician's position: The clinician is standing by the patient to observe the movement.

Command to patient: 'Bend your elbow so that your hand moves towards your shoulder.'

The elbow has to move through its full range of movement – full extension to full flexion.

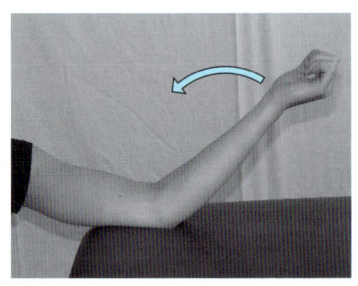

Fig 5.12 Oxford muscle grading for the elbow flexors – Grade 3. The elbow is moving from full extension to full flexion (the hand is moving towards the shoulder).

Grade 4 – 'Full ROM against minimal resistance'

Patient's position: The patient is positioned in sitting, with their arm supported on a table or plinth; their shoulder is in 90° of abduction, with the elbow fully extended and the forearm supinated.

Clinician's position: The clinician is standing by the patient, stabilizing their upper arm, applying a minimal resistance to the distal forearm.

Command to patient: 'Bend your elbow so that your hand moves towards your shoulder against the minimal resistance.'

The elbow has to move through its full range of movement – full extension to full flexion.

Clinical tip: Use the length of lever arm principle to make sure you can apply a consistent resistance to the limb. Ask the patient to start slowly so they can appreciate the amount of resistance.

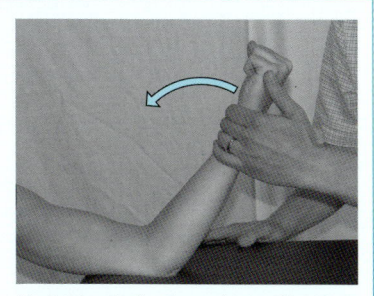

Fig 5.13 Oxford muscle grading for the elbow flexors – Grades 4 and 5. The elbow is moving from full extension to full flexion (the hand is moving towards the shoulder).

Grade 5 – 'Full ROM against maximal resistance'

Patient's position: The patient is positioned in sitting, with their arm supported on a table or plinth; their shoulder is in 90° of abduction, elbow fully extended and their forearm supinated (see Fig. 5.13).

Clinician's position: The clinician is standing by the patient, stabilizing their upper arm, providing a maximal resistance to the distal forearm.

Command to patient: 'Bend your elbow so that your hand moves towards your shoulder against the maximal resistance.'

The elbow has to move through its full range of movement – full extension to full flexion.

Clinical tip: Use the length of lever arm principle to make sure you can apply a consistent resistance to the limb. Ask the patient to start slowly so they can appreciate the amount of resistance.

Supinators

Grade 0 – 'No contraction' and Grade 1 – 'Flicker of a contraction'

Patient's position: The patient is positioned in sitting, with their arm supported on a table or plinth and their forearm in pronation.

Clinician's position: The clinician is standing by the patient, palpating the lateral border of the forearm and the biceps brachii muscle.

Command to patient: 'Try and make the muscles on this part of your arm tighten/turn your hand over.'

Clinical tip: Closely observing and feeling the muscle is essential in enabling the clinician to pick up on even the smallest flicker of a contraction.

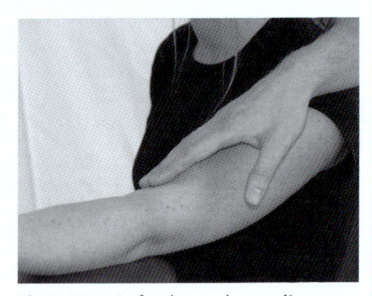

Fig 5.14 Oxford muscle grading for the elbow supinators – Grades 0 and 1.

Grade 2 – 'Full ROM with the effects of gravity eliminated'

This test is difficult to perform with the effects of gravity eliminated and therefore it is blended with Grade 3.

Patient's position: The patient is positioned in sitting, with their arm supported on a table or plinth and their forearm in pronation.

Clinician's position: The clinician is standing by the patient to observe the movement.

Command to patient: 'Try and move your forearm so that your hand turns over as far as you can.'

The elbow has to move through its full range of movement – full pronation to full supination.

Clinical tip: Ensure the upper arm is stabilized, otherwise the patient may perform lateral rotation of the shoulder.

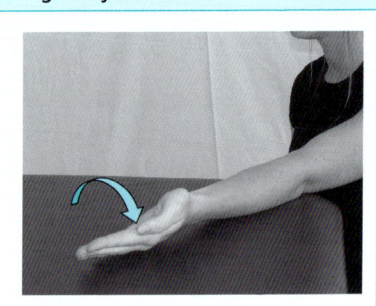

Fig 5.15 Oxford muscle grading for the elbow supinators – Grade 2. The forearm has moved from full pronation to full supination (the palm of the hand has moved from facing down to facing up).

Measurement

Grade 3 – 'Full ROM against the effects of gravity'

This test is difficult to perform against the effects of gravity.

Patient's position: The patient is positioned in sitting, with their arm supported on a table or plinth and their forearm in pronation.

Clinician's position: The clinician is standing by the patient to observe the movement.

Command to patient: 'Try and move your forearm so that your hand turns over as far as you can.'

The elbow has to move through its full range of movement – full pronation to full supination.

Clinical tip: Ensure the upper arm is stabilized, otherwise the patient may perform lateral rotation of the shoulder.

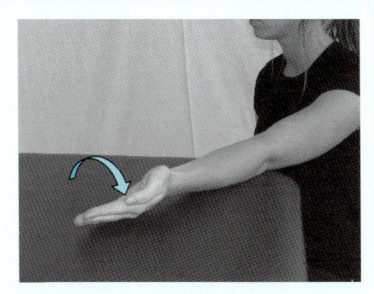

Fig 5.16 Oxford muscle grading for the elbow supinators – Grade 3. The forearm has moved from full pronation to full supination (the palm of the hand has moved from facing down to facing up).

Grade 4 – 'Full ROM against minimal resistance'

Patient's position: The patient is positioned in sitting, with their arm supported on a table or plinth and their forearm in pronation.

Clinician's position: The clinician is sitting by the patient, applying a minimal resistance to the dorsal aspect of the hand, resisting supination.

Command to patient: 'Try and move your forearm so that your hand turns over as far as you can, against the minimal resistance.'

The elbow has to move through its full range of movement – full pronation to full supination.

Clinical tip: Use the length of lever arm principle to make sure you can apply a consistent resistance to the limb. Ask the patient to start slowly so they can appreciate the amount of resistance.

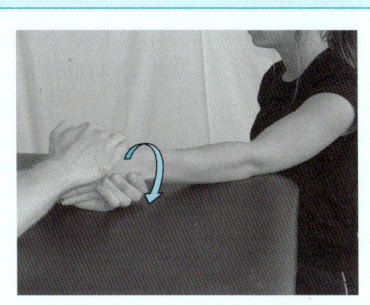

Fig 5.17 Oxford muscle grading for the elbow supinators – Grades 4 and 5. The forearm is moving from full pronation to full supination (the palm of the hand moving from facing down to facing up).

THE ELBOW JOINT

Grade 5 – 'Full ROM against maximal resistance'

Patient's position: The patient is positioned in sitting, their arm supported on a table or plinth and their forearm in pronation (see Fig. 5.17).

Clinician's position: The clinician is sitting by the patient, applying a maximal resistance to the dorsal aspect of the hand, resisting supination.

Command to patient: 'Try and move your forearm so that your hand turns over as far as you can, against the maximal resistance.'

The elbow has to move through its full range of movement – full pronation to full supination.

Clinical tip: Use the length of lever arm principle to make sure you can apply a consistent resistance to the limb. Ask the patient to start slowly so they can appreciate the amount of resistance.

Pronators

Grade 0 – 'No contraction' and Grade 1 – 'Flicker of a contraction'

Patient's position: The patient is positioned in sitting, their arm supported on a table or plinth and their forearm in pronation.

Clinician's position: The clinician is standing by the patient, palpating the muscle of pronator teres on the anterior/medial aspect of the forearm.

Command to patient: 'Try and make the muscles on this part of your arm tighten.'

Clinical tip: Closely observing and feeling the muscle is essential in enabling the clinician to pick up on even the smallest flicker of a contraction.

Pronator teres can be palpated on the medial border of the cubital fossa, between the medial epicondyle of the humerus and the middle of the radius.

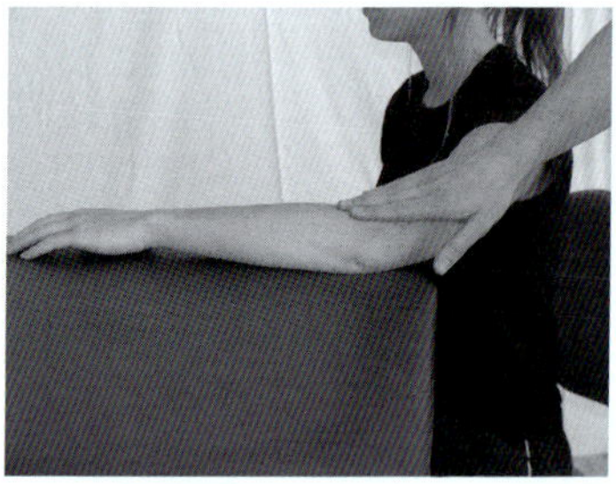

Fig 5.18 Oxford muscle grading for the elbow pronators – Grades 0 and 1.

Measurement

Grade 2 – 'Full ROM with the effects of gravity eliminated'

This test is difficult to perform with the effects of gravity eliminated, therefore it is blended with Grade 3.

Patient's position: The patient is positioned in sitting, their arm supported on a table or plinth and their forearm in supination.

Clinician's position: The clinician is standing by the patient to observe the movement.

Command to patient: 'Try and move your forearm so that your hand turns over as far as you can.'

The elbow has to move through its full range of movement – full supination to full pronation.

Clinical tip: Ensure the upper arm is stabilized, otherwise the patient may perform medial rotation of the shoulder.

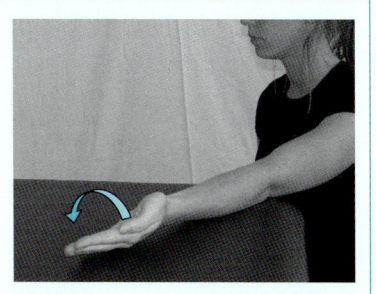

Fig 5.19 Oxford muscle grading for the elbow pronators – Grade 2/3. The forearm is moving from full supination to full pronation (the palm of the hand is moving from facing up to facing down).

Grade 3 – 'Full ROM against the effects of gravity'

This test is difficult to perform against the effects of gravity.

Patient's position: The patient is positioned in sitting, their arm supported on a table or plinth and their forearm in supination.

Clinician's position: The clinician is standing by the patient to observe the movement.

Command to patient: 'Try and move your forearm so that your hand turns over as far as you can.'

The elbow has to move through its full range of movement – full supination to full pronation.

Clinical tip: Ensure the upper arm is stabilized, otherwise the patient may perform medial rotation of the shoulder.

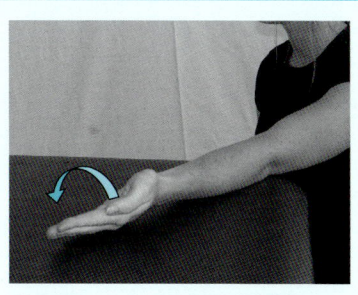

Fig 5.20 Oxford muscle grading for the elbow pronators – Grade 3. The forearm is moving from full supination to full pronation (the palm of the hand is moving from facing up to facing down).

THE ELBOW JOINT

Grade 4 – 'Full ROM against minimal resistance'

Patient's position: The patient is positioned in sitting, their arm supported on a table or plinth and their forearm in supination.

Clinician's position: The clinician is standing by the patient, providing a minimal resistance to the dorsal aspect of the hand, resisting pronation.

Command to patient: 'Try and move your forearm so that your hand turns over as far as you can, against the minimal resistance.'

The elbow has to move through its full range of movement – full supination to full pronation.

Clinical tip: Use the length of lever arm principle to make sure you can apply a consistent resistance to the limb. Ask the patient to start slowly so they can appreciate the amount of resistance.

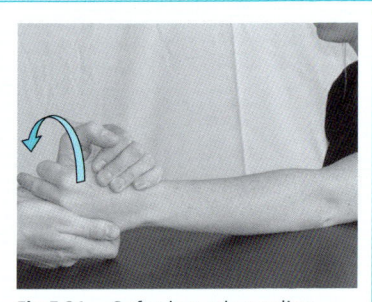

Fig 5.21 Oxford muscle grading for the elbow pronators – Grades 4 and 5. The forearm is moving from full supination to full pronation (the palm of the hand is moving from facing up to facing down).

Grade 5 – 'Full ROM against maximal resistance'

Patient's position: The patient is positioned in sitting, their arm supported on a table or plinth and their forearm in supination (see Fig. 5.21).

Clinician's position: The clinician is sitting by the patient, providing a maximal resistance to the dorsal aspect of the hand, resisting pronation.

Command to patient: 'Try and move your forearm so that your hand turns over as far as you can, against the maximal resistance.'

The elbow has to move through its full range of movement – full supination to full pronation.

Clinical tip: Use the length of lever arm principle to make sure you can apply a consistent resistance to the limb. Ask the patient to start slowly so they can appreciate the amount of resistance.

CHAPTER 6

The wrist/carpal joints

ANATOMY 149
  The wrist (radiocarpal) joint 149
  Bony landmarks to be palpated 150
  Ligaments 150
  Muscles 151
    Flexors 151
    Extensors 152
    Abductors/radial deviators 153
    Adductors/ulnar deviators 154
MEASUREMENT 155
  Range of movement 155
    Flexion 155
    Extension 156
    Adduction/ulnar deviation 157
    Abduction/radial deviation 158
    Observational/reflective checklist 160
  Muscle strength: Oxford muscle grading 161
    Extensors 161
    Flexors 163
    Adductors/ulnar deviators 165
    Abductors/radial deviators 167
  Joint girth 169
    Wrist 169
  Grip strength 170
    The hand-held dynamometer 170

ANATOMY

The wrist (radiocarpal) joint

1. It is a synovial ellipsoid joint.
2. It is formed between the distal surfaces of the radius and articular disc, and the scaphoid, lunate and triquetral of the proximal row of the carpal bones.
3. The capsular ligaments are the dorsal radiocarpal, palmar radiocarpal and palmar ulnocarpal ligaments.
4. The wrist joint has collateral ligaments – the radial and ulnar collateral carpal ligaments.

5. The movements that take place are flexion, extension, abduction (radial deviation) and adduction (ulnar deviation).

BONY LANDMARKS TO BE PALPATED

The radius – styloid process and dorsal tubercle.
The ulna – head of ulna and ulnar styloid process.
The carpus – pisiform, hook of hamate, tubercle of scaphoid and tubercle of trapezium.

LIGAMENTS

Table 6.1

\	\	\	\
The ligaments of the radiocarpal joint			
Ligament	Origin	Insertion	Limitation to movement
Ulnar collateral	Ulnar styloid process	Base of the pisiform and the triquetral	Abduction or radial deviation
Radial collateral	Tip of the radial styloid process	Lateral side of the scaphoid and lateral side of the trapezium	Adduction or ulnar deviation
Dorsal radiocarpal	Posterior edge of the distal end of the radius	Posterior surface of the lunate, scaphoid and triquetral	Flexion of the radiocarpal joint
Palmar radiocarpal	Anterior edge of the distal end of the radius	Anterior edge of the proximal row of carpal bones	Extension of the radiocarpal joint
Palmar ulnocarpal	Articular disc and ulnar styloid process	Anterior surface of the proximal row of carpal bones	Extension of the radiocarpal joint

Anatomy

MUSCLES
Flexors

Table 6.2

The flexors of the wrist				
Muscle	Origin	Insertion	Nerve supply	Action(s)
Flexor carpi ulnaris	Common flexor origin – medial epicondyle of the humerus	Hook of hamate, base of the 5th metacarpal	Ulnar nerve C7, 8	Flexion of the hand at the wrist
Flexor carpi radialis	Common flexor origin – medial epicondyle of the humerus	Palmar surface of the 2nd and 3rd metacarpals	Median nerve C6, 7	Flexion of the hand at the wrist
Palmaris longus	Common flexor origin – medial epicondyle of the humerus	Flexor retinaculum and the palmar aponeurosis	Median nerve C8	Flexion of the hand at the wrist
Flexor digitorum superficialis	Common flexor origin – medial epicondyle of the humerus. The ulnar collateral ligament and the anterior border of the radius	Palmar surface, base of the middle phalanx of the medial four fingers	Median nerve C7, 8, T1	Wrist flexion and flexion of the MCP and PIP joints
Flexor digitorum profundus	The upper three-quarters of the anterior and medial surfaces of the ulna	Base of the palmar surface of the distal phalanx of the medial four fingers	Anterior interosseous branch of the median nerve C7, 8, T1	Flexion of the DIP joints and flexion of the wrist joint
Flexor pollicis longus	Anterior surface of the radius, anterior surface of the interosseous membrane	Palmar surface of the base of the distal phalanx of the thumb	Anterior interosseous branch of the median nerve C7, 8, T1	Flexion of the interphalangeal joint of the thumb, and flexion of the wrist
MCP – metacarpophalangeal joints PIP – proximal interphalangeal joints DIP – distal interphalangeal joints CMC – carpometacarpal joint (thumb)				

Extensors

Table 6.3

The extensors of the wrist				
Muscle	Origin	Insertion	Nerve supply	Action(s)
Extensor carpi radialis longus	Anterior part of the lateral supracondylar ridge of the humerus	Posterior surface of the base of the 2nd metacarpal	Radial nerve C6, 7	Extension of the wrist
Extensor carpi radialis brevis	Common extensor origin of the lateral epicondyle of the humerus	Posterior surface of the base of the 3rd metacarpal	Posterior interosseous branch of the radial nerve C6, 7	Extension of the wrist, can produce abduction (radial deviation) when working with FCR
Extensor carpi ulnaris	Common extensor origin of the lateral epicondyle of the humerus	Medial side of the base of the 5th metacarpal	Posterior interosseous branch of the radial nerve C7, 8	Extension of the wrist
Extensor digitorum	Common extensor origin of the lateral epicondyle of the humerus	Base of the middle phalanx, dorsal aspect of the medial four fingers	Posterior interosseous branch of the radial nerve C7, 8	Extension of the MCP joints, also extension of the wrist
Extensor indicis	Posterior surface of the ulna and adjacent interosseous membrane	Dorsal digital expansion of the little finger	Posterior interosseous branch of the radial nerve C7, 8	Assists extensor digitorum and extends the wrist
Extensor digiti minimi	Common extensor origin of the lateral epicondyle of the humerus	Dorsal digital expansion of the little finger	Posterior interosseous branch of the radial nerve C7, 8	Extension of the MCP joints of the little finger and extension of the wrist

(table continues)

Anatomy

Table 6.3 (continued)

Muscle	Origin	Insertion	Nerve supply	Action(s)
Extensor pollicis longus	Lateral part of the middle third, posterior surface of the ulna and adjacent interosseous membrane	Dorsal surface of the base of the distal phalanx of the thumb	Posterior interosseous branch of the radial nerve C7, 8	Extension of all the joints of the thumb and extension and abduction of the wrist
Extensor pollicis brevis	Middle part of the posterior surface of the radius and adjacent interosseous membrane	Dorsal surface of the base of the proximal phalanx	Posterior interosseous branch of the radial nerve C7, 8	Extension of the CMC and MCP joints of the thumb and assists in extension and abduction of the wrist

MCP – metacarpophalangeal joints
CMC – carpometacarpal joint (thumb)
FCR – flexor carpi radialis

Abductors/radial deviators

Table 6.4

The abductors/radial deviators of the wrist				
Muscle	Origin	Insertion	Nerve supply	Action(s)
Extensor carpi radialis longus	Anterior part of the lateral supracondylar ridge of the humerus	Posterior surface of the base of the 2nd metacarpal	Radial nerve C6, 7	Extension and abduction of the wrist
Extensor carpi radialis brevis	Common extensor origin of the lateral epicondyle of the humerus	Posterior surface of the base of the 3rd metacarpal	Posterior interosseous branch of the radial nerve C6, 7	Extension of the wrist; can produce abduction when working with flexor carpi radialis
Flexor carpi radialis	Common flexor origin – medial epicondyle of the humerus	Palmar surface of the 2nd and 3rd metacarpals	Median nerve C6, 7	Flexion and abduction of the hand at the wrist

THE WRIST/CARPAL JOINTS

Adductors/ulnar deviators

Table 6.5

The adductors/ulnar deviators of the wrist				
Muscle	Origin	Insertion	Nerve supply	Action(s)
Extensor carpi ulnaris	Common extensor origin of the lateral epicondyle of the humerus	Medial side of the base of the 5th metacarpal	Posterior interosseous branch of the radial nerve C7, 8	Extension and adduction of the wrist
Flexor carpi ulnaris	Common flexor origin – medial epicondyle of the humerus	Hook of hamate, base of the 5th metacarpal	Ulnar nerve C7, 8	Flexion and adduction of the hand at the wrist

MEASUREMENT

RANGE OF MOVEMENT
Flexion

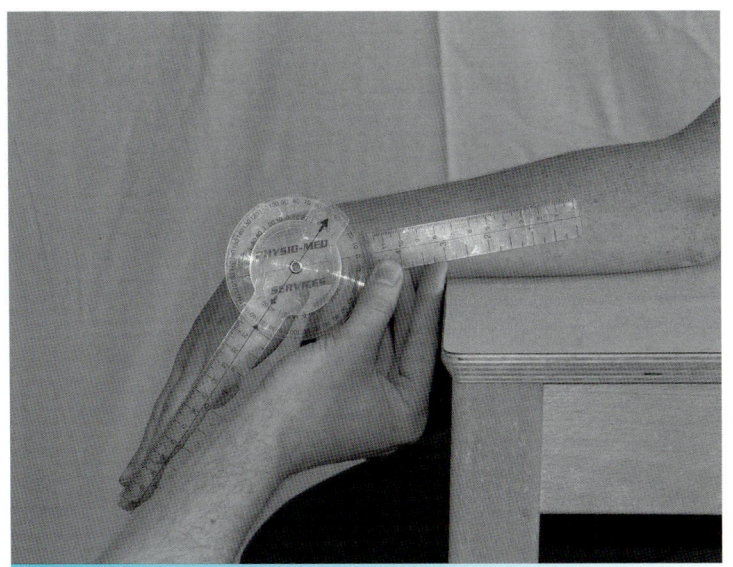

Fig 6.1 Goniometric measurement of wrist flexion.

Starting position: The patient is positioned in sitting, their forearm resting on a table in pronation and their wrist in a neutral position. The hand is over the end of the table.
Stabilization: The clinician stabilizes the forearm if necessary.
Goniometer axis: The axis of the goniometer is placed at the level of the ulnar styloid process.
Stationary arm: This is parallel to the long axis of the ulna.
Moveable arm: This is parallel to the long axis of the 5th metacarpal.
Command to patient: 'Move your hand downwards as far as you can.'
End position: The wrist is flexed to the limit of motion.
Trick movements: Ensure that no wrist deviation occurs as the hand is flexed.

NB: It may be necessary to reposition the stationary and moveable arms of the goniometer prior to taking the reading, as they may have moved when the patient flexed their wrist.

Extension

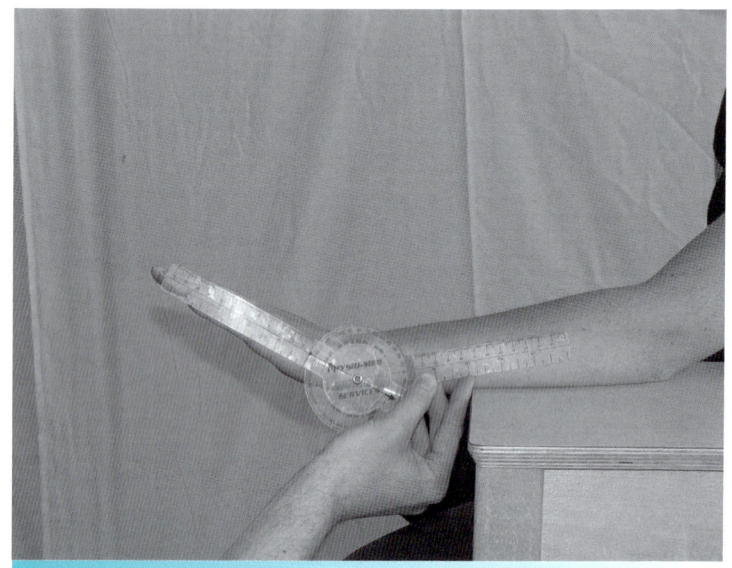

Fig 6.2 Goniometric measurement of wrist extension.

Starting position: The patient is positioned in sitting, their forearm resting on a table in pronation and their wrist in a neutral position. The hand is over the end of the table.
Stabilization: The clinician stabilizes the forearm if necessary.
Goniometer axis: The axis of the goniometer is placed at the level of the ulnar styloid process.
Stationary arm: This is parallel to the long axis of the ulna.
Moveable arm: This is parallel to the long axis of the 5th metacarpal.
Command to patient: 'Move your hand upwards as far as you can.'
End position: The wrist is extended to the limit of motion.

> *Clinical tip*
> Ensure that no wrist deviation occurs as the hand is extended.

> NB: It may be necessary to reposition the stationary and moveable arms of the goniometer prior to taking the reading, as they may have moved when the patient extended their wrist.

Adduction/ulnar deviation

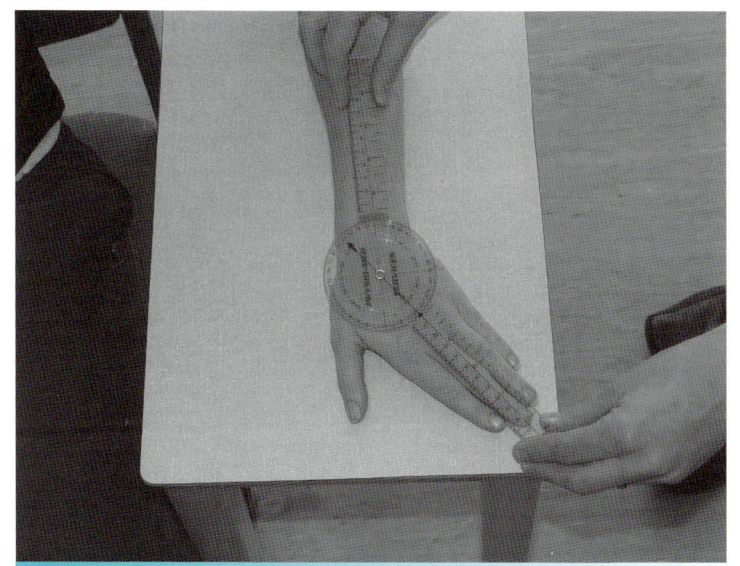

Fig 6.3 Goniometric measurement of wrist adduction/ulnar deviation.

Starting position: The patient is positioned in sitting, forearm pronated, their hand resting on a table.
Stabilization: The clinician stabilizes the forearm.
Goniometer axis: The axis of the goniometer is placed on the dorsal aspect of the wrist over the capitate bone.
Stationary arm: This is along the mid-line of the forearm.
Moveable arm: This is parallel to the long axis of the shaft of the 3rd metacarpal.
Command to patient: 'Move your hand outwards as far as you can.'
End position: The wrist is adducted/ulnar deviated to the limit of motion.

Ensure that the wrist is not moved into flexion or extension as the patient adducts/abducts to each side.

Clinical tip
To find the capitate bone, follow the shaft of the 3rd metacarpal proximally on the dorsal surface of the hand. At the end of the metacarpal you will feel the proximal head. After that your finger will slide onto a square(ish) flat structure, which is the capitate bone.

Abduction/radial deviation

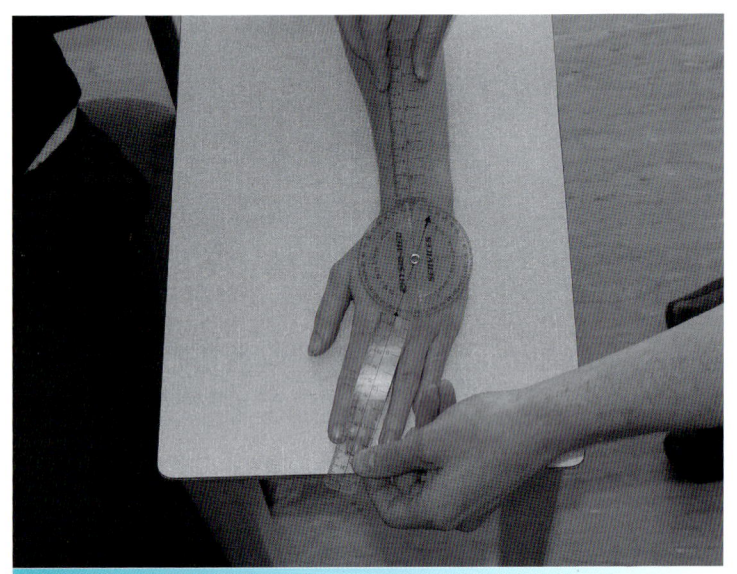

Fig 6.4 Goniometric measurement of wrist abduction/radial deviation.

Starting position: The patient is positioned in sitting, forearm pronated, their hand resting on a table.
Stabilization: The clinician stabilizes the forearm.
Goniometer axis: The axis of the goniometer is placed on the dorsal aspect of the wrist over the capitate bone.
Stationary arm: This is along the mid-line of the forearm.
Moveable arm: This is parallel to the long axis of the shaft of the 3rd metacarpal.
Command to patient: 'Move your hand in towards you as far as you can.'
End position: The wrist is abducted to the limit of motion.

> Ensure that the wrist is not moved into flexion or extension as the patient abducts/radial deviates.

Measurement

Notes

Treatment record

Observational/reflective checklist

Observation		Y/N	Comments
Introduction and preparation for the skill	Was the treatment area properly prepared for the patient, e.g. pillow, blanket, safe environment, etc.?		
	Did the therapist introduce him/herself?		
	Was the patient comfortable?		
	Was the patient adequately exposed/draped?		
	Was an explanation of the procedure given?		
	Was the explanation clear and succinct?		
	Was consent obtained?		
Performing the skill	Was the plinth set at the correct height?		
	Was the therapist's posture compromised?		
	Did the therapist identify the joint and other relevant bony landmarks?		
	Was the goniometer correctly aligned?		
	Was the reading of the joint range of movement accurate?		
	Did the therapist compare both sides of the body?		
Safe and effective performance of the technique	Was the procedure carried out with due care and attention?		
How would you rate the proficiency in the overall performance of the skill?	Excellent		
	Very good		
	Good		
	Satisfactory		
	Borderline		
	Fail		

Measurement

MUSCLE STRENGTH: OXFORD MUSCLE GRADING

Extensors

Grade 0 – 'No contraction' and Grade 1 – 'Flicker of a contraction'

Patient's position: The patient is positioned in sitting, their forearm resting on a table and in pronation.

Clinician's position: The clinician is sitting or standing by the patient, palpating the extensor surface of the forearm.

Command to patient: 'Try and make the muscles on this part of your arm tighten/try and lift your fingers upwards.'

Clinical tip: Closely observing and feeling the muscle is essential in enabling the clinician to pick up on even the smallest flicker of a contraction.

The lateral epicondyle of the humerus is the 'common extensor origin', where several of the wrist and hand extensor muscles have their origin.

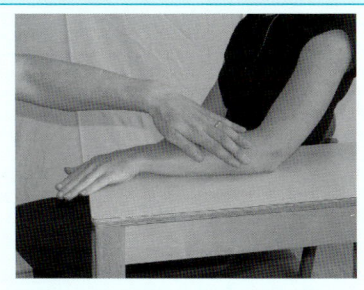

Fig 6.5 Oxford muscle grading for the wrist extensors – Grades 0 and 1.

Grade 2 – 'Full ROM with the effects of gravity eliminated'

Patient's position: The patient is positioned in sitting, their arm supported on a table. Their forearm is in the mid-pronation/supination position and their wrist is in full flexion.

Clinician's position: The clinician is sitting or standing by the patient, supporting the weight of the hand and stabilizing the forearm.

Command to patient: 'Try and move your hand backwards as far as you can.'

The wrist has to move through its full range of movement – full flexion to full extension.

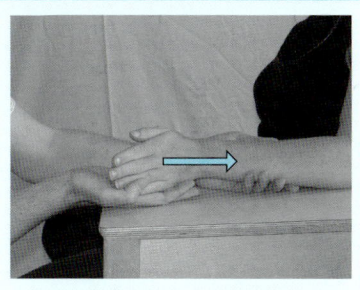

Fig 6.6 Oxford muscle grading for the wrist extensors – Grade 2. The wrist is moving from full flexion to full extension (the dorsum of hand is moving backwards).

THE WRIST/CARPAL JOINTS

Grade 3 – 'Full ROM against the effects of gravity'

Patient's position: The patient is positioned in sitting, their arm supported on a table. Their hand is over the end of the table, in full flexion.

Clinician's position: The clinician is sitting or standing by the patient to observe the movement.

Command to patient: 'Try and lift your hand up so that your fingers are pointing towards the ceiling, as far as you can.'

The wrist has to move through its full range of movement – full flexion to full extension.

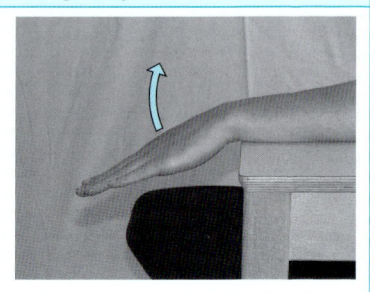

Fig 6.7 Oxford muscle grading for the wrist extensors – Grade 3. The wrist is moving from full flexion to full extension (the dorsum of the hand is moving upwards).

Grade 4 – 'Full ROM against minimal resistance'

Patient's position: The patient is positioned in sitting, their arm supported on a table. Their hand is over the end of the table, in full flexion.

Clinician's position: The clinician is standing or sitting by the patient, applying a minimal resistance to the dorsal surface of the hand.

Command to patient: 'Try and lift your hand up so that your fingers are pointing towards the ceiling, against the minimal resistance.'

The wrist has to move through its full range of movement – full flexion to full extension.

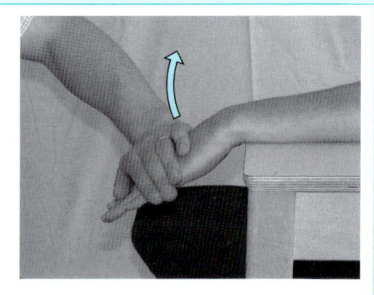

Fig 6.8 Oxford muscle grading for the wrist extensors – Grades 4 and 5. The wrist is moving from full flexion to full extension (the dorsum of the hand is moving upwards).

Grade 5 – 'Full ROM against maximal resistance'

Patient's position: The patient is positioned in sitting, their arm supported on a table. Their hand is over the end of the table, in full flexion (see Fig. 6.8).

Clinician's position: The clinician is standing or sitting by the patient, applying a maximal resistance to the dorsal surface of the hand.

Command to patient: 'Try and lift your hand up so that your fingers are pointing towards the ceiling, against the maximal resistance.'

The wrist has to move through its full range of movement – full flexion to full extension.

Measurement

Flexors

Grade 0 – 'No contraction' and Grade 1 – 'Flicker of a contraction'

Patient's position: The patient is positioned in sitting, their arm supported on a table and their forearm in pronation.

Clinician's position: The clinician is standing or sitting by the patient, palpating the flexor surface of the forearm, especially the medial epicondyle of the humerus.

Command to patient: 'Try and make the muscles on this part of your arm tighten/try and move your fingers downwards.'

Clinical tip: Closely observing and feeling the muscle is essential in enabling the clinician to pick up on even the smallest flicker of a contraction.

Clinical tip: The medial epicondyle of the humerus is the 'common extensor origin', where several flexors of the wrist and hand take their origin.

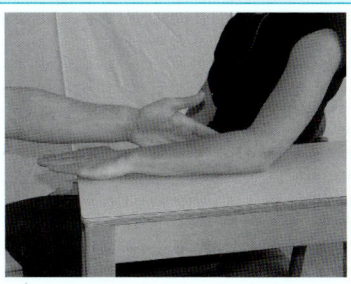

Fig 6.9 Oxford muscle grading for the wrist flexors – Grades 0 and 1.

Grade 2 – 'Full ROM with the effects of gravity eliminated'

Patient's position: The patient is positioned in sitting, their arm supported on a table. Their forearm is in the mid-pronation/supination position and their wrist is in full extension.

Clinician's position: The clinician is standing or sitting by the patient, supporting the weight of their hand and stabilizing the forearm.

Command to patient: 'Try and move your hand inwards as far as you can.'

The wrist has to move through its full range of movement – full extension to full flexion.

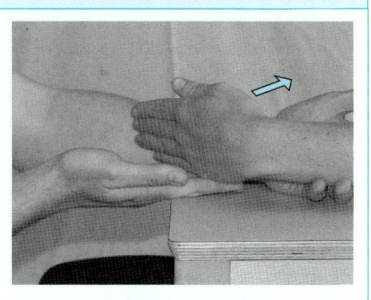

Fig 6.10 Oxford muscle grading for the wrist flexors – Grade 2. The wrist is moving from full extension to full flexion (the palm of the hand is moving inwards).

THE WRIST/CARPAL JOINTS

Grade 3 – 'Full ROM against the effects of gravity'

Patient's position: The patient is positioned in sitting, their supinated arm supported on a table. Their hand is over the end of the table, in full extension.

Clinician's position: The clinician is standing or sitting by the patient, observing the movement.

Command to patient: 'Try and bend your wrist up as far as you can, so that your fingers are pointing towards the ceiling.'

The wrist is moving from full extension to full flexion.

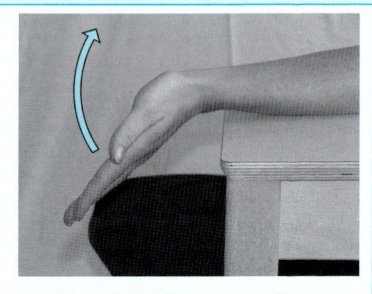

Fig 6.11 Oxford muscle grading for the wrist flexors – Grade 3. The wrist is moving from full extension to full flexion (the palm of the hand is moving upwards).

Grade 4 – 'Full ROM against minimal resistance'

Patient's position: The patient is positioned in sitting, their supinated arm supported on a table. Their hand is over the end of the table, in full extension.

Clinician's position: The clinician is standing or sitting by the patient, applying a minimal resistance to the palmar surface of the hand.

Command to patient: 'Try and bend your wrist up as far as you can, against the minimal resistance, so that your fingers are pointing towards the ceiling.'

The wrist is moving from full extension to full flexion.

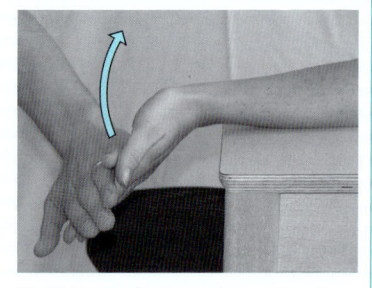

Fig 6.12 Oxford muscle grading for the wrist flexors – Grades 4 and 5. The wrist is moving from full extension to full flexion (the palm of the hand is moving upwards).

Grade 5 – 'Full ROM against maximal resistance'

Patient's position: The patient is positioned in sitting, their supinated arm supported on a table. Their hand is over the edge of the table, in full extension (see Fig. 6.12).

Clinician's position: The clinician is standing or sitting by the patient, applying a maximal resistance to the palmar surface of the hand.

Command to patient: 'Try and bend your wrist up as far as you can, against the maximal resistance, so that your fingers are pointing towards the ceiling.'

The wrist is moving from full extension to full flexion.

Measurement

Adductors/ulnar deviators

Grade 0 – 'No contraction' and Grade 1 – 'Flicker of a contraction'

Patient's position: The patient is positioned in sitting, their arm supported on a table and their forearm in supination.

Clinician's position: The clinician is standing or sitting by the patient, palpating the medial border of their forearm for the flexor carpi ulnaris muscle.

Command to patient: 'Try and make the muscles on this part of your arm tighten/move your hand away from your body.'

Clinical tip: Closely observing and feeling the muscle is essential in enabling the clinician to pick up on even the smallest flicker of a contraction.

The tendon of flexor carpi ulnaris can be felt just proximal to the pisiform.

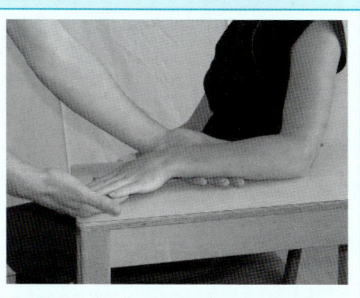

Fig 6.13 Oxford muscle grading for the wrist adductors/ulnar deviators – Grades 0 and 1.

Grade 2 – 'Full ROM with the effects of gravity eliminated'

Patient's position: The patient is positioned in sitting, their arm supported on a table. Their forearm is in pronation and fully abducted.

Clinician's position: The clinician is standing or sitting by the patient, supporting the weight of their hand and stabilizing the forearm.

Command to patient: 'Try and move your hand outwards, away from your body as far as you can.'

The wrist has moved from full abduction to full adduction.

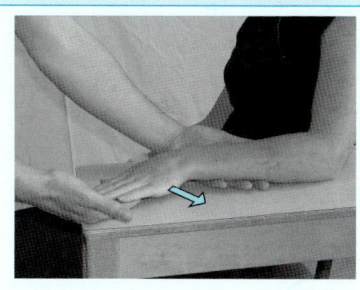

Fig 6.14 Oxford muscle grading for the wrist adductors/ ulnar deviators – Grade 2. The wrist is moving from full abduction to full adduction (the hand is moving away from the body).

THE WRIST/CARPAL JOINTS

Grade 3 – 'Full ROM against the effects of gravity'

Patient's position: This is a very difficult movement for the patient to achieve. Their shoulder/arm must be supported in approximately 45° of shoulder flexion, their arm fully medially rotated and their elbow in extension. Their wrist, which is over the end of the table, is in neutral and their hand is in full abduction.

Clinician's position: The clinician is standing or sitting by the patient to observe the movement.

Command to patient: 'Move your hand upwards towards the ceiling as far as you can.'

The wrist moves from full abduction to full adduction.

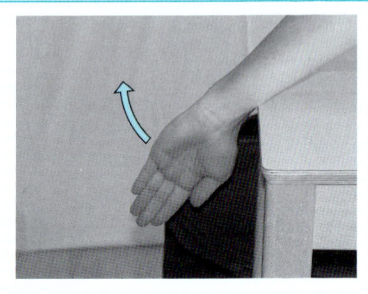

Fig 6.15 Oxford muscle grading for the wrist adductors/ulnar deviators – Grade 3. The wrist is moving from full abduction to full adduction (the palm of the hand is moving up towards the ceiling).

Grade 4 – 'Full ROM against minimal resistance'

Patient's position: The patient is positioned in sitting, their pronated arm supported on a table. Their hand is over the end of the table and their wrist is in full abduction.

Clinician's position: The clinician is sitting by the patient, stabilizing their forearm and applying a minimal resistance to the medial surface of the hand.

Command to patient: 'Try to move your hand outwards as far as you can against the minimal resistance.'

The wrist is moving from full abduction to full adduction.

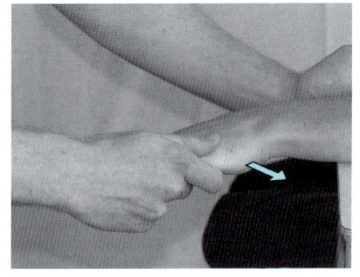

Fig 6.16 Oxford muscle grading for the wrist adductors/ulnar deviators – Grades 4 and 5. The wrist is moving from full abduction to full adduction (the hand is moving away from the body).

Grade 5 – 'Full ROM against maximal resistance'

Patient's position: The patient is positioned in sitting, their pronated arm supported on a table. Their hand is over the end of the table and their wrist is in full abduction (see Fig. 6.16).

Clinician's position: The clinician is sitting by the patient, stabilizing the forearm and applying a maximal resistance to the medial surface of the hand.

Command to patient: 'Try to move your hand outwards as far as you can against the maximal resistance.'

The wrist moves from full abduction to full adduction.

Measurement

Abductors/radial deviators

Grade 0 – 'No contraction' and Grade 1 – 'Flicker of a contraction'

Patient's position: The patient is positioned in sitting, their arm supported on a table and their forearm in pronation.

Clinician's position: The clinician is sitting or standing by the patient, palpating the lateral border of their forearm for the flexor carpi radialis muscle/tendon.

Command to patient: 'Try and make the muscles on this part of your arm tighten/try and move your hand in towards your body.'

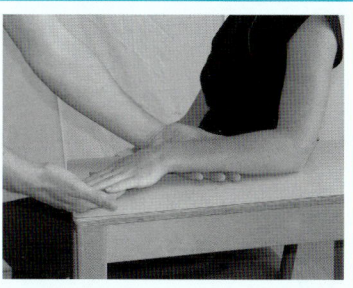

Fig 6.17 Oxford muscle grading for the wrist abductors/radial deviators – Grades 0 and 1.

Clinical tip: Closely observing and feeling the muscle is essential in enabling the clinician to pick up on even the smallest flicker of a contraction.

The tendon of flexor carpi radialis can be felt on the anterior aspect of the wrist, it being the most lateral tendon.

Grade 2 – 'Full ROM with the effects of gravity eliminated'

Patient's position: The patient is positioned in sitting, their arm supported on a table. Their forearm is in pronation and fully adducted.

Clinician's position: The clinician is sitting or standing by the patient, supporting the weight of their hand and stabilizing the forearm.

Command to patient: 'Try and move your wrist so that your thumb moves inwards towards your body as far as you can.'

The wrist is moving from full adduction (ulnar deviation) to full abduction (radial deviation).

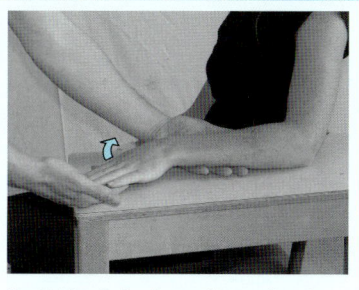

Fig 6.18 Oxford muscle grading for the wrist abductors/radial deviators – Grade 2. The wrist is moving from full adduction to full abduction (the hand is moving in towards the body).

THE WRIST/CARPAL JOINTS

Grade 3 – 'Full ROM against the effects of gravity'

Patient's position: The patient is positioned in sitting, their arm supported on a table and their wrist and hand off the end of the table. Their wrist is in adduction/ulnar deviation and their forearm is in the mid-supination/pronation position.

Clinician's position: The clinician is sitting or standing by the patient, stabilizing their forearm and observing the movement.

Command to patient: 'Try and move your wrist so that your thumb moves up towards the ceiling as far as you can.'

The wrist is moving from full adduction (ulnar deviation) to full abduction (radial deviation).

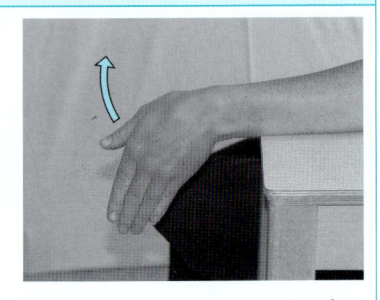

Fig 6.19 Oxford muscle grading for the wrist abductors/radial deviators – Grade 3. The wrist moves from full adduction (ulnar deviation) to full abduction (radial deviation).

Grade 4 – 'Full ROM against minimal resistance'

Patient's position: The patient is positioned in sitting, their arm supported on a table and their wrist and hand off the end of the table. Their wrist is in adduction/ulnar deviation and their forearm is in pronation.

Clinician's position: The clinician is sitting or standing by the patient, stabilizing their forearm, applying a minimal resistance to the lateral aspect of the hand.

Command to patient: 'Try and move your wrist against the minimal resistance, so that your thumb moves in towards your body.'

The wrist moves from full adduction (ulnar deviation) to full abduction (radial deviation).

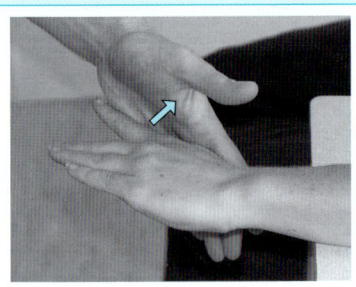

Fig 6.20 Oxford muscle grading for the wrist abductors/radial deviators – Grades 4 and 5. The wrist moves from full adduction (ulnar deviation) to full abduction (radial deviation).

Grade 5 – 'Full ROM against maximal resistance'

Patient's position: The patient is positioned in sitting, their arm supported on a table and their wrist and hand off the end of the table. Their wrist is in adduction/ulnar deviation, their forearm in pronation (see Fig. 6.20).

Clinician's position: The clinician is sitting or standing by the patient, stabilizing their forearm, applying a maximal resistance to the lateral aspect of the hand.

Command to patient: 'Try and move your wrist as far as you can, against the maximal resistance, so that your thumb moves in towards your body.'

The wrist moves from full adduction (ulnar deviation) to full abduction (radial deviation).

JOINT GIRTH
Wrist

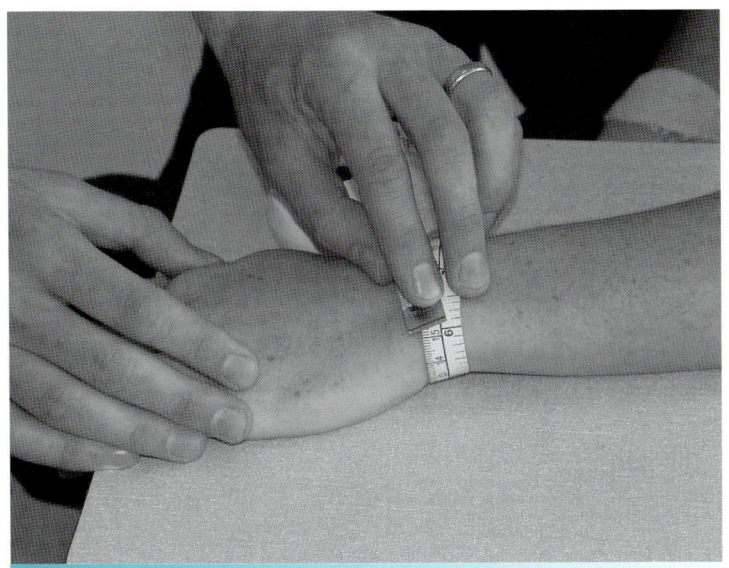

Fig 6.21 Measurement of the girth of the wrist joint.

The wrist joint line is identified by drawing a line between the radial styloid process and the ulnar styloid process.

Patient's position: The patient is positioned in sitting with their arm supported on a table.

Method: The joint girth may be measured by taking a circumferential measurement with a tape measure around the joint line.

Repeat the procedure three times and produce an average reading. Repeat the procedure on the other limb to compare the results.

Points to note:
The state of the tape measure – is it stretched or twisted?
The muscles must be relaxed.
Keep the tape measure straight.
Measure consistently, using the top or bottom aspect of the tape each time. Are you measuring in inches or centimetres?

GRIP STRENGTH
The hand-held dynamometer

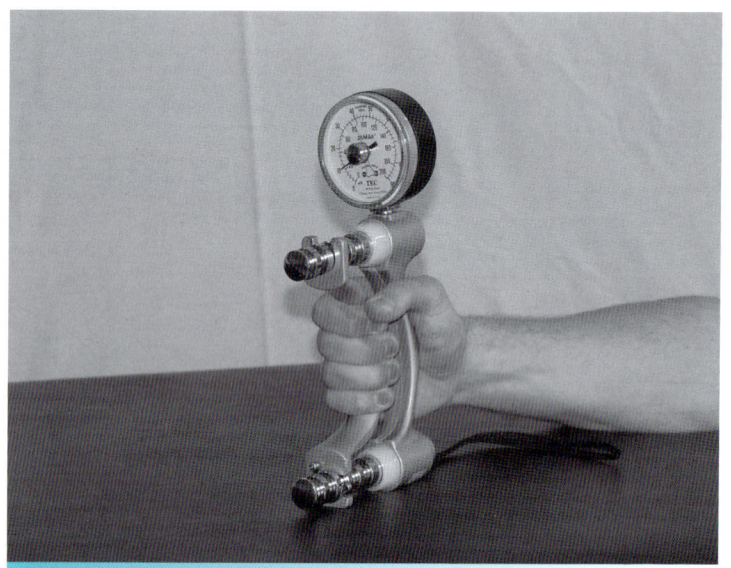

Fig 6.22 Testing grip strength with a hand-held dynamometer.

To measure grip strength a Jamar dynamometer may be used. It consists of a sealed hydraulic system, with a gauge calibrated in pounds or kilograms.
Patient's position: The patient is comfortably seated, their shoulder adducted and in neutral rotation. Their elbow is in 90° of flexion, with their forearm and wrist in the neutral position. The patient comfortably holds the instrument in their hand.

Make sure the red peak-hold needle is turned to 0 prior to testing. The dynamometer is generally set to the second handle position.

Command to patient: The clinician tells the patient to squeeze the handle as hard as they can by saying – 'Squeeze as hard as you can ... harder ... harder ... relax'.

The red peak-hold needle has to be turned anti-clockwise to return to 0.

Three trials are recorded, with a 2–3 minute rest between each trial. The score taken is the average of the three trials.

Measurement

Notes

Treatment record

172 THE WRIST/CARPAL JOINTS

Notes

Treatment record

CHAPTER 7

The hand

ANATOMY 173
    The thumb 173
    The fingers 173
  Bony landmarks to be palpated 173
  Ligaments 174
  Muscles 174
    Extensors 174
    Flexors 175
    Abductors, adductors and opposers 175
MEASUREMENT 176
  Range of movement – CMC joint of the thumb 176
    Abduction 176
    Flexion/extension 177
  Range of movement – MCP joint of the thumb 178
    Flexion 178
  Range of movement – IP joint of the thumb 179
    Flexion 179
  Range of movement – MCP joint of the finger 180
    Flexion 180
    Abduction 181
  Range of movement – PIP joint of the finger 182
    Flexion/extension 182
  Range of movement – DIP joint of the finger 183
    Flexion/extension 183
    Observational/reflective checklist 185

ANATOMY

The thumb

1. The carpometacarpal (CMC) joint of the thumb is a synovial saddle joint.
2. It is an articulation between the trapezium and the base of the first metacarpal.
3. The two surfaces are reciprocally concavoconvex.
4. A loose but strong fibrous capsule encloses the joint.
5. Movements of flexion, extension, abduction, adduction and opposition occur at this joint.

The fingers

1. The metacarpophalangeal (MCP) joint is synovial condyloid joint.
2. It is an articulation between the head of the metacarpal and the base of the proximal phalanx.
3. A loose fibrous capsule surrounds the joint.
4. There are strong collateral ligaments on either side of the joint.

5. The movements that take place at this joint are flexion, extension, abduction and adduction.
6. The interphalangeal (IP) joints are synovial hinge joints.
7. Each finger has three phalanges, therefore there is a proximal (PIP) and distal (DIP) interphalangeal joint.
8. A loose fibrous capsule surrounds the joint.
9. There are strong collateral ligaments on either side of the joint.
10. The movements that take place at the joint are flexion and extension.

BONY LANDMARKS TO BE PALPATED

The carpus – scaphod, lunate, triquetral, pisiform, trapezium, trapezoid, capitate, hamate. The metacarpals and phalanges.

LIGAMENTS

Table 7.1

Ligaments of the hand			
Ligament	Origin	Insertion	Limitation to movement
Radial carpometacarpal ligament	Lateral surface of the trapezium	Lateral surface of the first metacarpal	
Anterior oblique ligament	Anterior surface of the trapezium	Medial side of the first metacarpal	Taut posterior oblique ligament
Posterior oblique ligament	Posterior surface of the trapezium	Medial side of the first metacarpal	Taut anterior oblique ligament

MUSCLES
Extensors

Table 7.2

The extensors of the thumb				
Muscle	Origin	Insertion	Nerve supply	Action(s)
Extensor pollicis longus	Middle third of the posterior surface of the ulna and interosseous membrane	Dorsal surface of the distal phalanx of the thumb	Posterior interosseous branch of the radial nerve C7, 8	Extension and radial deviation of the wrist. Extension of all the thumb joints
Extensor pollicis brevis	Middle part of the posterior surface of the radius and interosseous membrane	Dorsal surface of the base of the proximal phalanx	Posterior interosseous branch of the radial nerve C7, 8	Extension and radial deviation of the wrist. Extension of the carpometacarpal and metacarpophalangeal (MCP) joints of the thumb

Anatomy

Flexors

Table 7.3

The flexors of the thumb

Muscle	Origin	Insertion	Nerve supply	Action(s)
Flexor pollicis longus	Upper anterior surface of the radius and interosseous membrane	Palmar surface of the distal phalanx of the thumb	Anterior interosseous branch of the median nerve C8, T1	Flexion of the wrist joint. Flexion of the interphalangeal and metacarpophalangeal joints of the thumb. Vital in all gripping activities
Flexor pollicis brevis	Flexor retinaculum, tubercle of the trapezium, capitate and trapezoid	Radial side of the base of the proximal phalanx of the thumb	Median nerve T1	Flexion of the carpometacarpal and metacarpophalangeal joints of the thumb. It also produces medial rotation of the thumb

Abductors, adductors and opposers

Table 7.4

The abductors, adductors and opposers of the thumb

Muscle	Origin	Insertion	Nerve supply	Action(s)
Abductor pollicis longus	Upper, posterior surface of the ulna, middle third of the posterior surface of the radius and the interosseous membrane	Radial side of the base of the first metacarpal	Posterior interosseous branch of the radial nerve C7, 8	Working with abductor pollicis brevis it abducts the thumb. Working with the extensors it extends the thumb at the CMC joint. Working by itself it moves the thumb into a mid-extended and abducted position
Abductor pollicis brevis	Flexor retinaculum, and tubercles of scaphoid and trapezium	Radial side of proximal phalanx of the thumb	Median nerve T1	Abduction of the thumb at the CMC and MCP joints

(*table continues*)

Table 7.4 (continued)

Muscle	Origin	Insertion	Nerve supply	Action(s)
Opponens pollicis	Flexor retinaculum and tubercle of the trapezium	Lateral half of the anterior surface of the first metacarpal	Median nerve T1	Opposition of the thumb – abduction, medial rotation, and flexion and adduction of the CMC joint. This allows precise hand actions to take place
Palmaris brevis	Palmar aponeurosis and flexor retinaculum	The skin of the medial border of the hand	Ulnar nerve T1	This muscle wrinkles the skin on the ulnar side of the hand and assists the thumb in producing a good grip

MEASUREMENT

RANGE OF MOVEMENT – CARPOMETACARPAL (CMC) JOINT OF THE THUMB
Abduction

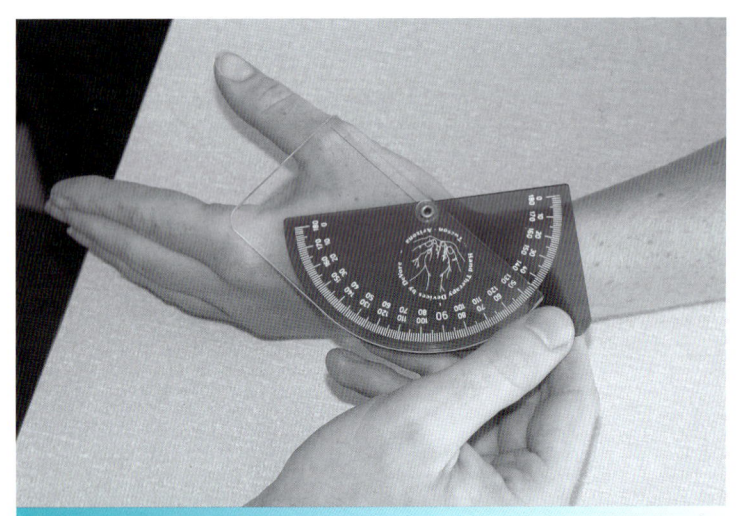

Fig 7.1 Goniometric measurement of the carpometacarpal joint of the thumb – abduction.

Starting position: The patient is positioned in sitting, their arm supported on a table. Their elbow is flexed, their forearm is in the

Measurement

mid-position, their wrist is in the anatomical position and the thumb maintains contact with the metacarpal of the index finger.
Goniometer axis: The axis of the goniometer is placed at the junction of the bases of the first and second metacarpal. (A small goniometer is required.)
Stationary arm: This is parallel to the longitudinal axis of the second metacarpal.
Moveable arm: This is parallel to the longitudinal axis of the first metacarpal. In the start position this will indicate 15–20°. Record as 0°.
End position: The thumb is abducted to the limit of motion (70°).

Flexion/extension

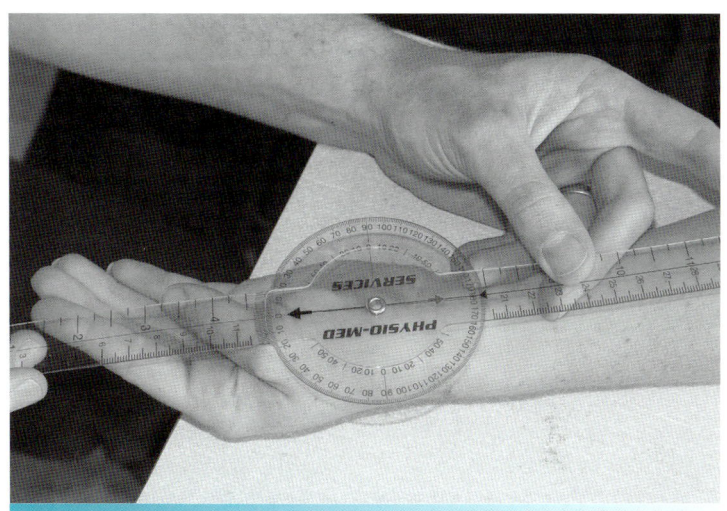

Fig 7.2 Goniometric measurement of the carpometacarpal joint of the thumb – flexion and extension.

Starting position: The patient is positioned in sitting, their arm supported on a table. Their elbow is flexed, their forearm is in supination and their wrist is in neutral.
Goniometer axis: The axis of the goniometer is placed over the CMC joint of the thumb. (A small goniometer is required.)
Stationary arm: This is parallel to the longitudinal axis of the radius.
Moveable arm: This is parallel to the longitudinal axis of the thumb metacarpal.
End position: Flexion – the thumb if flexed across palm (15°).
Extension – the thumb is extended away from the palm (20°).

RANGE OF MOVEMENT – METACARPOPHALANGEAL (MCP) JOINT OF THE THUMB
Flexion

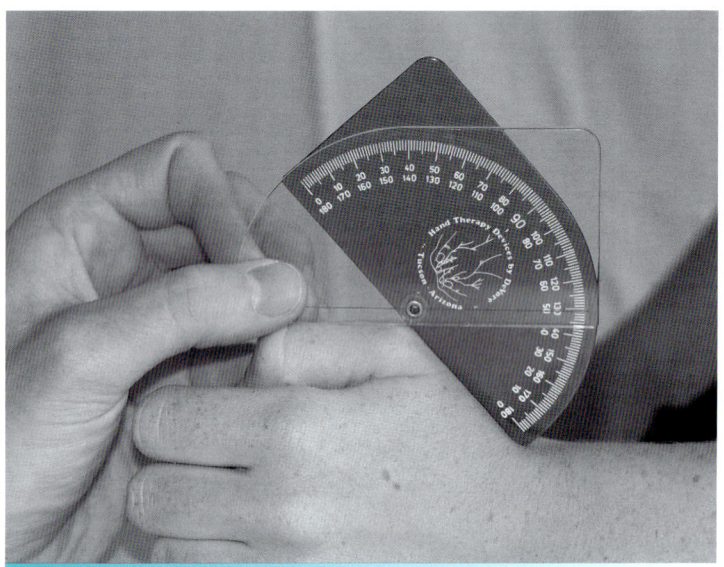

Fig 7.3 Goniometric measurement of finger metacarpophalangeal (MCP) flexion.

Starting position: The patient is positioned in sitting, their arm supported on a table. Their elbow is flexed, their forearm is in the mid-position and their wrist is slightly extended. The MCP joint being measured is in 0° of extension.
Stabilization: The clinician stabilizes the metacarpal.
Goniometer axis: The axis of the goniometer is placed over the dorsal aspect of the joint being measured. (A small goniometer is required.)
Stationary arm: This is parallel to the longitudinal axis of the shaft of the metacarpal.
Moveable arm: This is parallel to the longitudinal axis of the proximal phalanx.
End position: The MCP joint is flexed to the limit of motion.

> **Clinical tip**
> During the movement the interphalangeal (IP) joint is allowed to flex.

Measurement

RANGE OF MOVEMENT – INTERPHALANGEAL (IP) JOINT OF THE THUMB
Flexion

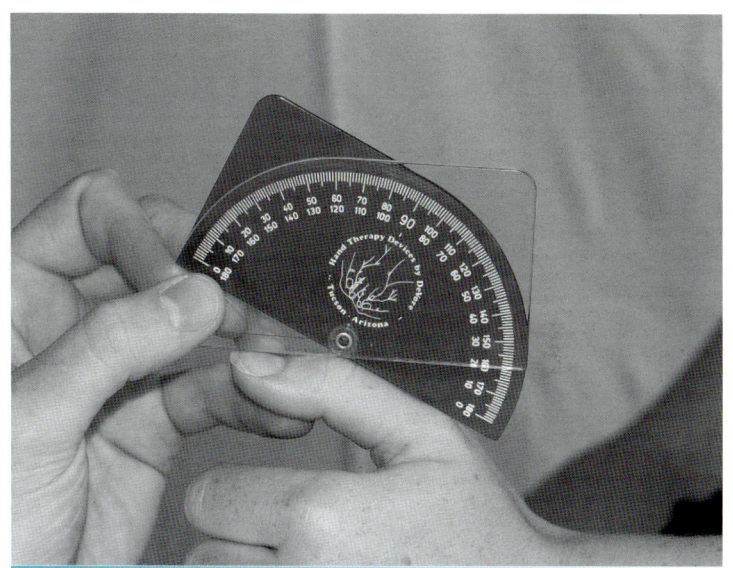

Fig 7.4 Goniometric measurement of thumb interphalangeal (IP) flexion.

Starting position: The patient is positioned in sitting, their arm supported on a table. Their elbow is flexed, their forearm is in the mid-position and their wrist is slightly extended. The IP joint being measured is in 0° of extension.
Stabilization: The clinician stabilizes the metacarpal.
Goniometer axis: The axis of the goniometer is placed over the dorsal aspect of the joint being measured.
Stationary arm: This is parallel to the longitudinal axis of the shaft of the proximal phalanx.
Moveable arm: This is parallel to the longitudinal axis of the distal phalanx.
End position: The thumb is flexed to the limit of motion.

RANGE OF MOVEMENT – METACARPOPHALANGEAL (MCP) JOINT OF THE FINGER
Flexion

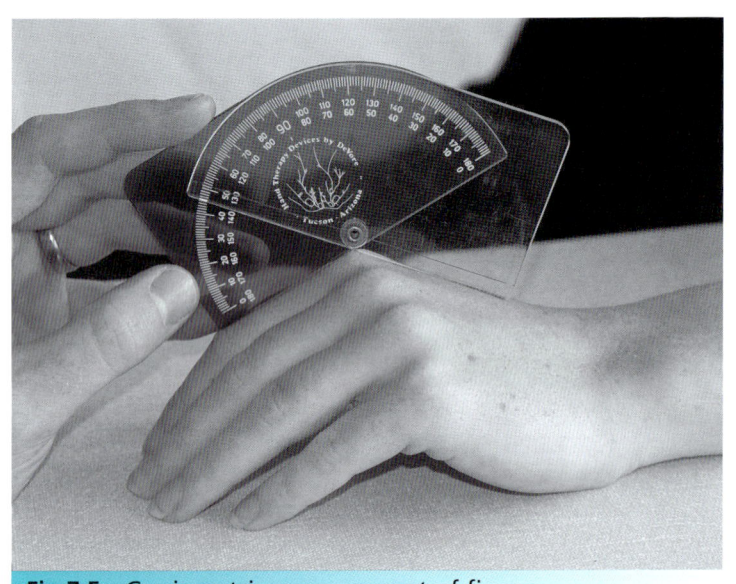

Fig 7.5 Goniometric measurement of finger metacarpophalangeal (MCP) flexion.

Starting position: The patient is positioned in sitting, their arm supported on a table. Their elbow is flexed, their forearm is in pronation and their wrist is extended. The MCP joint being measured is in 0° of extension.
Stabilization: The clinician stabilizes the metacarpal.
Goniometer axis: The axis of the goniometer is placed over the dorsal aspect of the joint being measured.
Stationary arm: This is parallel to the longitudinal axis of the shaft of the metacarpal.
Moveable arm: This is parallel to the longitudinal axis of the proximal phalanx.
End position: The MCP joint is flexed to the limit of motion.

> *Clinical tip*
> During the movement the proximal interphalangeal (PIP) joint is allowed to flex and the distal interphalangeal (DIP) joint remains in extension.

RANGE OF MOVEMENT – METACARPOPHALANGEAL (MCP) JOINT OF THE FINGER
Abduction

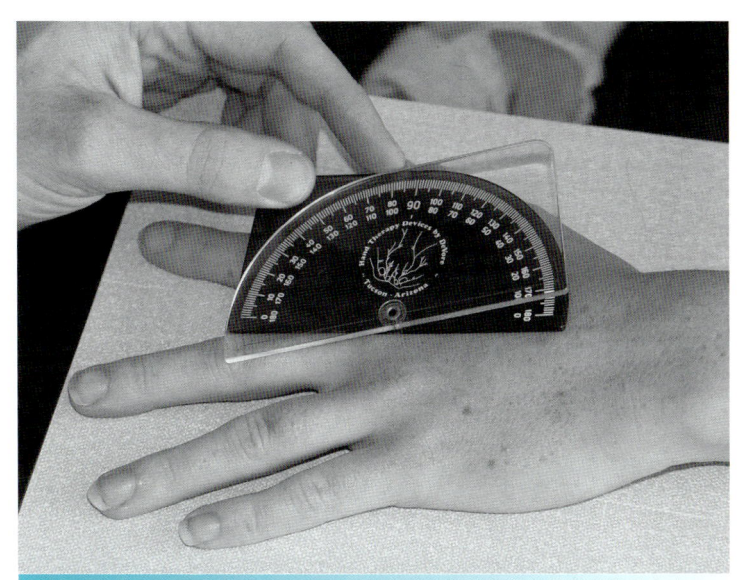

Fig 7.6 Goniometric measurement of finger metacarpophalangeal (MCP) abduction.

Starting position: The patient is positioned in sitting, their arm supported on a table. Their elbow is flexed, their forearm is in pronation and their wrist is in neutral.
Stabilization: The clinician stabilizes the metacarpals.
Goniometer axis: The axis of the goniometer is placed over the dorsal surface of the MCP joint being measured.
Stationary arm: This is parallel to the long axis of the shaft of the metacarpal.
Moveable arm: This is parallel to the long axis of the proximal phalanx.
End position: The finger is moved away from the mid-line.
Alternate method: The patient spreads his/her hand out on a page. The clinician draws round the hand. After the patient removes their hand, the clinician records the linear measurement between the mid-point of each finger.

THE HAND

RANGE OF MOVEMENT – PROXIMAL INTERPHALANGEAL (PIP) JOINT OF THE FINGER
Flexion/extension

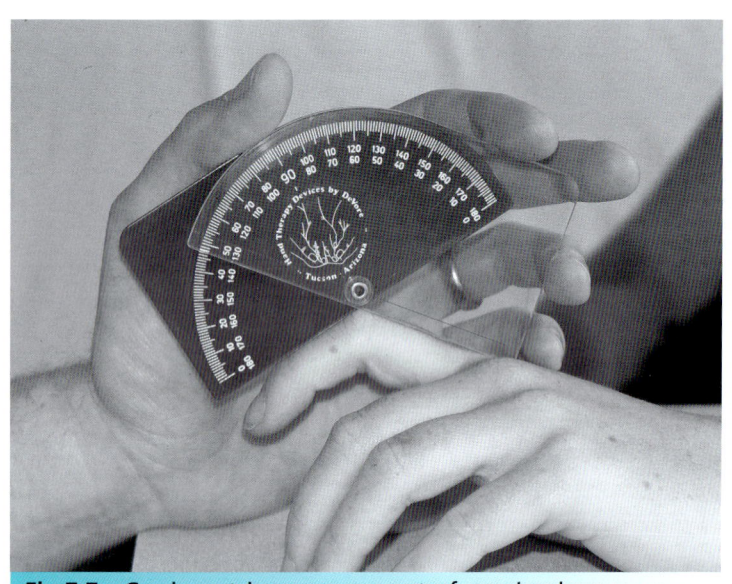

Fig 7.7 Goniometric measurement of proximal interphalangeal (PIP) flexion and extension.

Starting position: The patient is positioned in sitting, their arm supported on a table. Their elbow is flexed, their forearm is in pronation and their wrist and fingers are in extension (0° of extension at the MCP and IP joints).
Stabilization: The clinician stabilizes the phalanx, proximal to the joint being measured.
Goniometer axis: The axis of the goniometer is placed over the dorsal surface of the PIP joint being measured.
Stationary arm: This is parallel to the longitudinal axis of the proximal phalanx.
Moveable arm: This is parallel to the longitudinal axis of the middle phalanx.
End position: The PIP joint is flexed to the limit of motion.

RANGE OF MOVEMENT – DISTAL INTERPHALANGEAL (DIP) JOINT OF THE FINGER
Flexion/extension

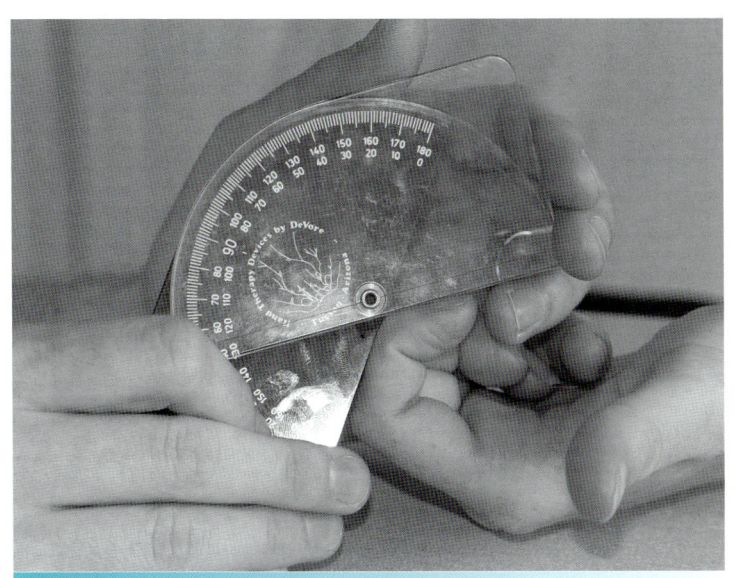

Fig 7.8 Goniometric measurement of distal interphalangeal (DIP) flexion and extension.

Starting position: The patient is positioned in sitting, their arm supported on a table. Their elbow is flexed, their forearm is in supination and their wrist and fingers are in extension (0° of extension at the MCP and IP joints).
Stabilization: The clinician stabilizes the phalanx, proximal to the joint being measured.
Goniometer axis: The axis of the goniometer is placed over the dorsal surface of the DIP joint being measured.
Stationary arm: This is parallel to the longitudinal axis of the middle phalanx.
Moveable arm: This is parallel to the longitudinal axis of the distal phalanx.
End position: The DIP joint is flexed to the limit of motion.

THE HAND

Notes

Treatment record

Observational/reflective checklist

Observational/reflective checklist			
Observation		Y/N	Comments
Introduction and preparation for the skill	Was the treatment area properly prepared for the patient, e.g. pillow, blanket, safe environment, etc.?		
	Did the therapist introduce him/herself?		
	Was the patient comfortable?		
	Was the patient adequately exposed/draped?		
	Was an explanation of the procedure given?		
	Was the explanation clear and succinct?		
	Was consent obtained?		
Performing the skill	Was the plinth set at the correct height?		
	Was the therapist's posture compromised?		
	Did the therapist identify the joint and other relevant bony landmarks?		
	Was the goniometer correctly aligned?		
	Was the reading of the joint range of movement accurate?		
	Did the therapist compare both sides of the body?		
Safe and effective performance of the technique	Was the procedure carried out with due care and attention?		
How would you rate the proficiency in the overall performance of the skill?	Excellent		
	Very good		
	Good		
	Satisfactory		
	Borderline		
	Fail		

Notes

Treatment record

CHAPTER

The spine

8

ANATOMY 187
   Ligaments 188
   Muscles 189
      Trunk flexors 189
      Trunk extensors 190
      Neck flexors 191
      Neck extensors 192
   Bony landmarks to be palpated 192
MEASUREMENT 192
   Range of movement 192
      Trunk flexion – lumbar spine 192
      Trunk extension – lumbar spine 193
      Trunk flexion/extension – lumbar spine 194
      Trunk lateral flexion (side flexion) 196
      Observational/reflective checklist 198
      Neck flexion using a tape measure 199

Measurement of neck flexion using an inclinometer 200
Neck flexion using an inclinometer 201
Neck extension using a tape measure 202
Neck extension using an inclinometer 203
Neck lateral flexion using a tape measure 204
Neck lateral flexion using an inclinometer 205
Neck rotation using a tape measure 206
Measurement of neck rotation using a compass goniometer 207

ANATOMY

1. The spine consists of 24 free vertebrae: 7 cervical, 12 thoracic and 5 lumbar.
2. Anteriorly, the vertebral bodies are bound by intervertebral discs.
3. The intervertebral discs are composed of fibrocartilage and comprise one-quarter of the total length of the vertebral column.

4. Individual discs are wedge shaped, in conformity with the curvature of the vertebral column in the region of the disc.
5. Therefore, curvatures in the cervical and lumbar regions are due to the greater anterior thickness of disc.
6. Shapes of disc: cervical – oval, thoracic – heart shaped, lumbar – kidney shaped. Posteriorly, the vertebral bodies are united by synovial, plane joints – zygapophyseal/facet joints. The shape and orientation of the joint surfaces vary in the three regions.
7. *In the cervical spine* the articular surfaces are flat and oval and lie in an oblique plane. Movements: flexion, extension, lateral flexion (side flexion) and rotation.
8. *In the thoracic spine* the articular surfaces on the superior processes project almost vertically. Movements: flexion, extension, lateral flexion and rotation.
9. *In the lumbar spine* there are strong articular processes that have a marked upwards and downwards projection. Movements: flexion, extension and lateral flexion.

LIGAMENTS

Table 8.1

The spinal ligaments			
Ligament	Origin	Insertion	Limitation to movement
Anterior longitudinal ligament (three dense layers of collagen)	Anterior aspect of the vertebral bodies – atlas	Sacrum	Extension
Posterior longitudinal ligament (two dense layers of collagen)	Posterior aspect of the vertebral bodies – axis	Sacrum	Flexion
Ligamentum flavum	Laminae above, from C1 to L5	Laminae below, from C1 to L5	Flexion
Supraspinous ligament	Spinous process above	Spinous process below	Flexion
Ligamentum nuchae	Spine of C7	External occipital protuberance	Flexion
Interspinous ligaments	Vertebral spine above	Vertebral spine below	Flexion

MUSCLES
Trunk flexors

Table 8.2

The flexors of the trunk

Muscle	Origin	Insertion	Nerve supply	Action(s)
Rectus abdominis	Symphysis pubis and pubic crest	Xiphoid process and costal cartilages of fifth, sixth and seventh ribs	Anterior primary rami of the lower six or seven thoracic nerves	Flexion and lateral flexion of the trunk
External oblique	Outer borders of lower eight ribs and their costal cartilages	Outer lip of the anterior two-thirds of the iliac crest, forming an aponeurosis, to fuse with the one from the opposite side at the linea alba. The lower free border, running between the anterior superior iliac spine and the pubic tubercle, forms the inguinal ligament	Lower six or seven thoracic nerves and first lumbar nerve	Flexion, lateral flexion and rotation of the trunk
Internal oblique	From the lateral two-thirds of the inguinal ligament, the anterior two-thirds of the iliac crest and from the thoracolumbar fascia	Inferior border of lower four ribs, an aponeurotic sheet which fuses with the one from the opposite side at the linea alba. The muscle arising from the inguinal ligament blends with the transversus abdominis to form the conjoint tendon	Lower six or seven thoracic nerves and first lumbar nerve	Flexion, lateral flexion and rotation of the trunk
Transversus abdominis	Lateral third of the inguinal ligament, anterior two-thirds of inner lip of iliac crest, thoracolumbar fascia and inner surface of lower six ribs and their costal cartilages	It forms an aponeurotic sheet which fuses with the aponeurosis of the internal oblique, eventually reaching the linea alba	Lower six or seven thoracic nerves and first lumbar nerve	Flexion, lateral flexion and rotation of the trunk

Anatomy 189

Trunk extensors

Table 8.3

The extensors of the trunk				
Muscle	Origin	Insertion	Nerve supply	Action(s)
Erector spinae	Spinous processes and supraspinous ligament T11 to L5, posterior sacral crest, sacrotuberous ligament, posterior part of the iliac crest			
Iliocostalis – lumborum	From the origin above	Lower six ribs	Adjacent primary rami	Extension, lateral flexion and rotation of the trunk
– thoracis	Lower six ribs	Upper six ribs		
– cervicis	Upper six ribs	Transverse processes of C4–C7		
Longissimus – thoracis	Transverse processes of lumbar vertebrae	Transverse processes of all thoracic vertebrae and lower ten ribs	Adjacent primary rami	Extension, lateral flexion and rotation of the trunk
– cervicis	Transverse processes of T1–T6	Transverse processes of C2–C6		
– capitis	Transverse processes of T1–T5 and articular processes of C4–C7	Mastoid process of the temporal bone		
Spinalis – thoracis	Spinous processes of T11–L2	Spinous processes of T1–T6	Adjacent primary rami	Extension, lateral flexion and rotation of the trunk
– cervicis – capitis	Both are poorly developed muscles and blend with adjacent muscles			

(*table continues*)

Anatomy

Table 8.3 (continued)

The extensors of the trunk				
Muscle	Origin	Insertion	Nerve supply	Action(s)
Quadratus lumborum	Iliolumbar ligament, adjacent iliac crest	Twelfth rib, transverse processes of the lumbar vertebrae	Anterior rami T12–L4	Extension and lateral flexion of the trunk
Multifidus	Sacrum, mamillary processes of the lumbar vertebrae, transverse processes of the thoracic vertebrae and the articular processes of the lower four or five cervical vertebrae	The muscle fibres are arranged in three layers as they pass upwards and medially to attach to the spinous processes of all the vertebrae from L5 to C2	Adjacent primary rami	Extension, lateral flexion and rotation of the trunk

Neck flexors

Table 8.4

The flexors of the neck				
Muscle	Origin	Insertion	Nerve supply	Action(s)
Sternomastoid	Anterior surface of the manubrium sterni and the upper surface of the medial third of the clavicle	Mastoid process of the temporal bone and the superior nuchal line of the occipital bone	Accessory nerve (eleventh cranial)	Flexion, lateral flexion and rotation of the neck
Scalenus anterior	Anterior tubercles of the transverse processes of C3–C6	Scalene tubercle of the first rib	Ventral rami C4, C5, C6	Flexion and lateral flexion of the neck

Neck extensors

Table 8.5

The extensors of the neck				
Muscle	Origin	Insertion	Nerve supply	Action(s)
Splenius capitis	Ligamentum nuchae and spinous processes C7–T4	Mastoid process of the temporal bone and adjacent superior nuchal line	Primary rami C3, C4, C5	Extension, lateral flexion and rotation of the neck
Erector spinae Longissimus capitis	Transverse processes of T1–T5 and articular processes of C4–C7	Mastoid process of the temporal bone		Extension and lateral flexion of the neck

BONY LANDMARKS TO BE PALPATED

Spinous processes in the cervical, thoracic and lumbar regions.
Transverse processes in cervical and thoracic regions. All the ribs.

MEASUREMENT

RANGE OF MOVEMENT

Trunk flexion – lumbar spine

Starting position: The patient is positioned in standing, with their feet shoulder-width apart. Their hands are resting on the anterior aspect of their thighs.

Command to patient: 'Slide your hands down the front of your legs as far as you can.'

End position: The patient slides their hands down the front of their thighs/legs to flex the trunk forwards (flexion).

Measurement: A tape measure is used to measure the distance between tip of the third digit and the floor. As the patient's spinal range of movement increases, this distance decreases.

Measurement 193

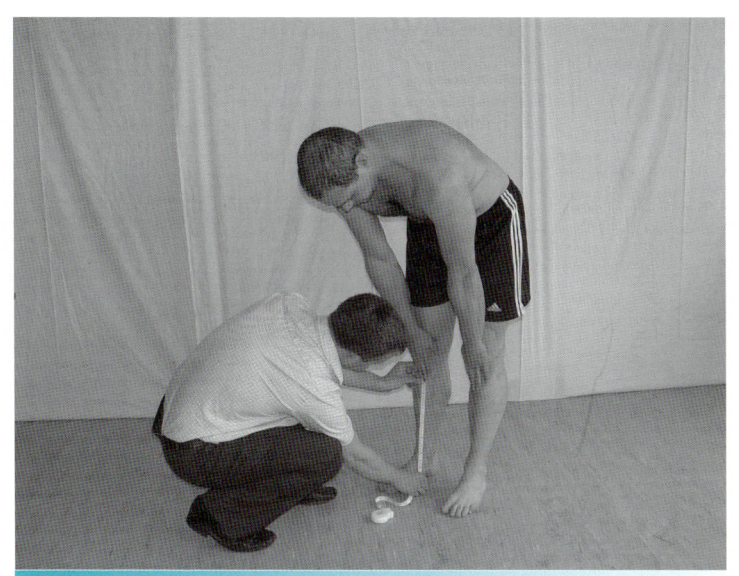

Fig 8.1 Measurement of trunk flexion using a tape measure.

Trunk extension – lumbar spine

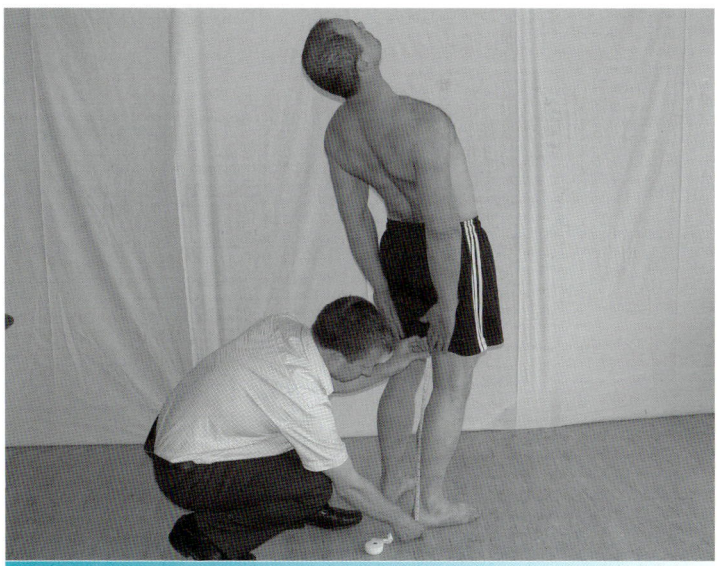

Fig 8.2 Measurement of trunk extension with a tape measure.

Starting position: The patient is positioned in standing, with their feet shoulder-width apart. Their hands are resting on the posterior aspect of their legs.
Command to patient: 'Slide your hands down the back of your legs as far as you can.'
End position: The patient slides their hands down the back of their thighs to extend the lumbar spine (extension).
Measurement: A tape measure is used to measure the distance between tip of the third digit and the floor. As the patient's spinal range of movement increases, this distance decreases.

Trunk flexion/extension – lumbar spine

This test is also known as the modified Schober test.

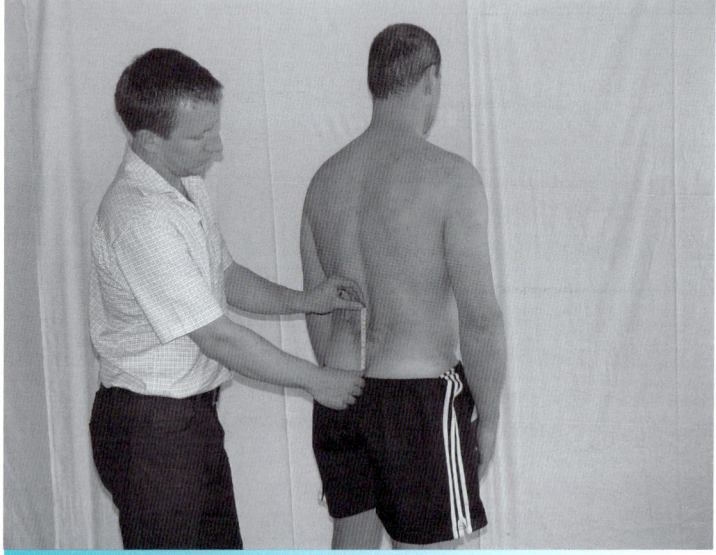

Fig 8.3 Measurement of spinal flexion using a tape measure.

Starting position: The patient is positioned in standing, with their feet shoulder-width apart. Their hands are resting on the anterior aspect of their thighs.
Measurement: Draw a line between the posterior superior iliac spines (PSISs). Use a tape measure to mark a point 10 cm above this line and another 5 cm below it. A measure is taken at the start position.

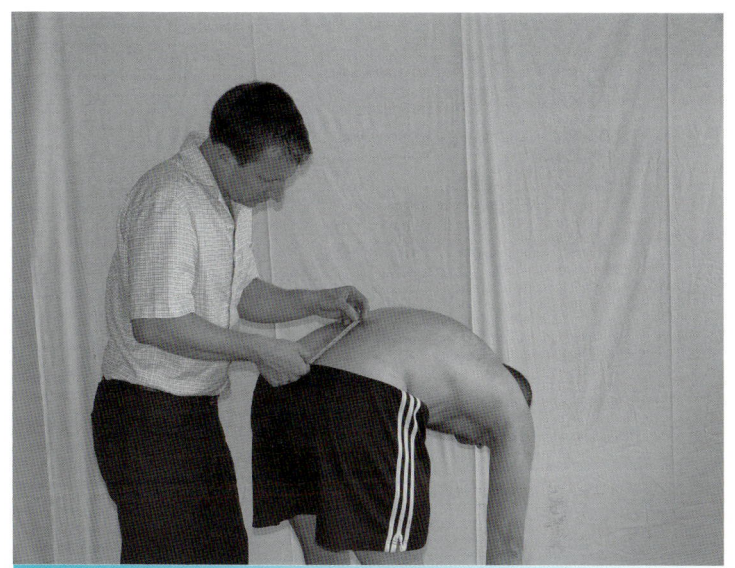

Fig 8.4 Measurement of spinal flexion.

Command to patient: 'Slide your hands down the front of your legs as far as you can.'

End position: The patient slides their hands down the front of their thighs/legs to flex the trunk forwards (flexion) to the limit of motion.

A measure is taken at the start position and at the limit of motion of flexion. The distance between the two measures is the lumbar flexion spinal range of movement. As the patient's spinal range of movement increases, this distance increases.

Trunk lateral flexion (side flexion)

Starting position: The patient is positioned in standing, with their feet shoulder-width apart. Their hands are resting on the lateral aspect of their legs.
Command to patient: 'Slide your hand down the side of your leg as far as you can.'
End position: The patient laterally flexes the trunk. They slide their hand down the side of their leg.
Measurement: A tape measure is used to measure the distance between the tip of the third digit and the floor.
Trick movement: Trunk flexion or extension.

Measure the range of movement to the opposite side.

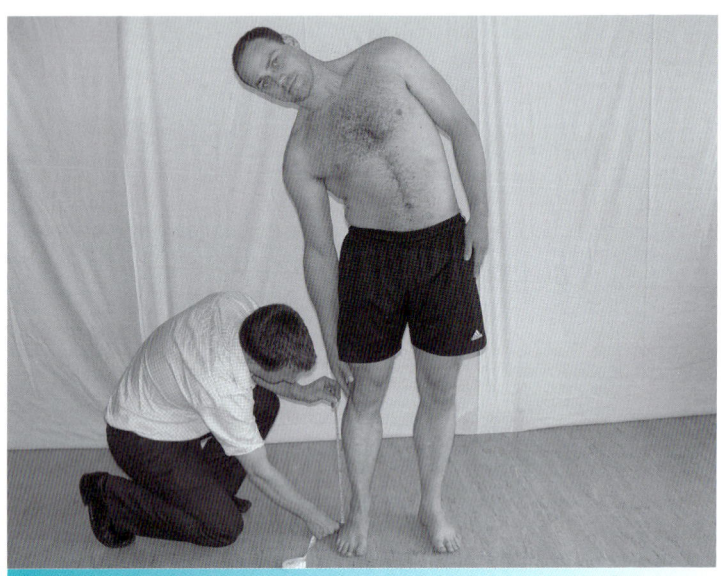

Fig 8.5 Measurement of trunk lateral flexion (side flexion) using a tape measure.

Measurement 197

Notes

Treatment record

Observational/reflective checklist

Observational/reflective checklist			
Observation		Y/N	Comments
Introduction and preparation for the skill	Was the treatment area properly prepared for the patient, e.g. pillow, blanket, safe environment, etc.?		
	Did the therapist introduce him/herself?		
	Was the patient comfortable?		
	Was the patient adequately exposed/draped?		
	Was an explanation of the procedure given?		
	Was the explanation clear and succinct?		
	Was consent obtained?		
Performing the skill	Was the therapist's posture compromised?		
	Did the therapist identify the joint and other relevant bony landmarks?		
	Was the tape measure correctly aligned?		
	Was the reading of the spinal movement accurate?		
Safe and effective performance of the technique	Was the procedure carried out with due care and attention?		
How would you rate the proficiency in the overall performance of the skill?	Excellent		
	Very good		
	Good		
	Satisfactory		
	Borderline		
	Fail		

Measurement 199

Neck flexion using a tape measure

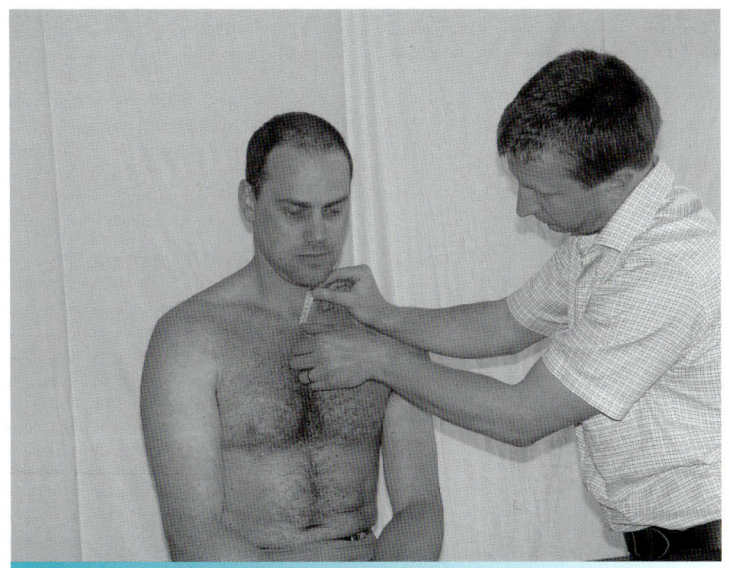

Fig 8.6 Measurement of neck flexion using a tape measure.

Starting position: The patient is positioned in sitting, head and neck in the anatomical position.
Command to patient: 'Move your chin down to your chest as far as you can.'
End position: The patient flexes the neck to the limit of motion – neck flexion.
Measurement: A tape measure is used to measure the distance between the tip of the chin and the suprasternal notch (flexion).
Trick movement: Mouth opening.

Measurement of neck flexion using an inclinometer

The cervical measurement system consists of a special head device, easily adjustable for each size of head, on to which are placed two separate inclinometers and a compass goniometer. These are positioned on the head apparatus so that neck flexion/extension, side flexion and rotation can be easily measured.

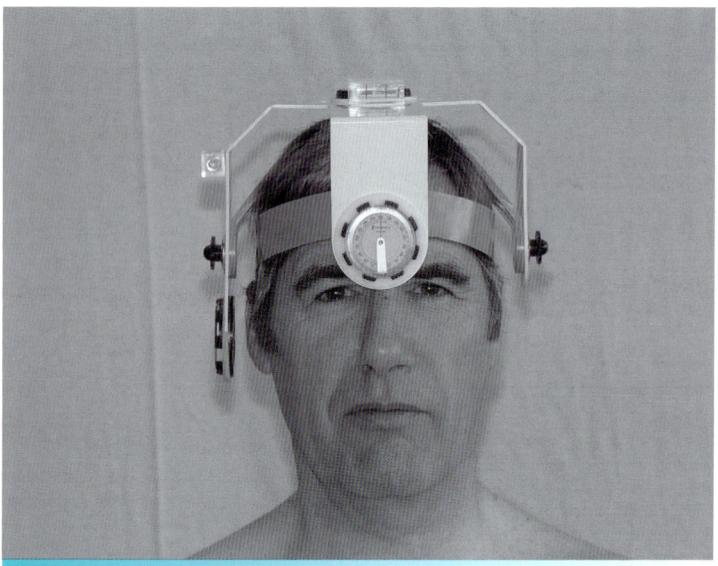

Fig 8.7 The inclinometer in situ on the head of the patient.

Starting position: The patient is positioned in sitting, head and neck in the anatomical position. Ensure that the measurement device is horizontal on the patient's head and the inclinometer should read zero.

Neck flexion using an inclinometer

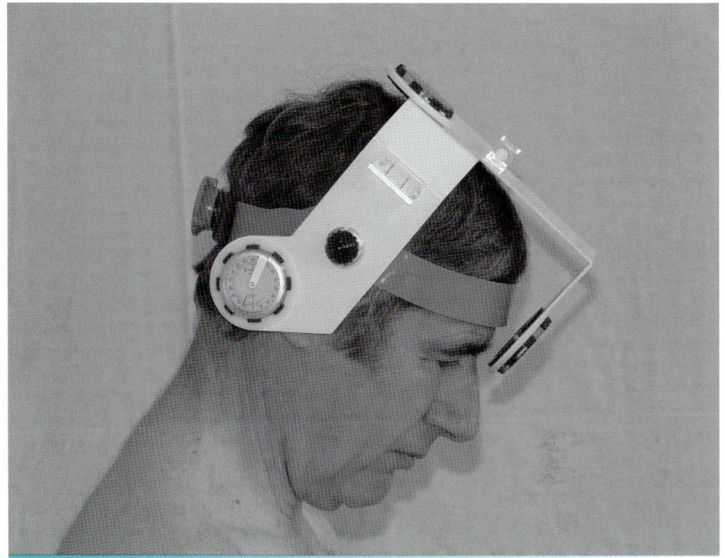

Fig 8.8 Measurement of neck flexion using an inclinometer.

Starting position: The patient is positioned in sitting, head and neck in the anatomical position.
Command to patient: 'Move your chin down to your chest as far as you can.'
End position: The patient flexes the neck to the limit of motion (chin to chest).

Neck extension using a tape measure

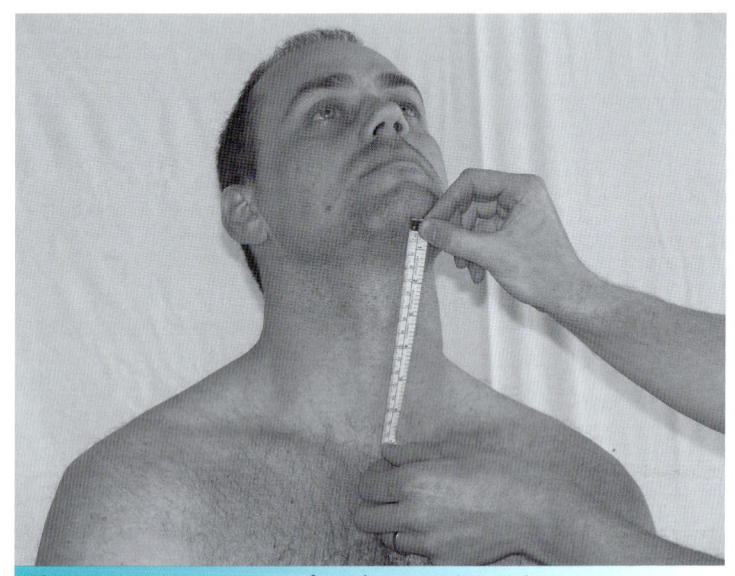

Fig 8.9 Measurement of neck extension using a tape measure.

Starting position: The patient is positioned in sitting, head and neck in the anatomical position.
Command to patient: 'Look up to the ceiling as far as you can.'
End position: The patient extends the neck to the limit of motion – neck extension.
Measurement: A tape measure is used to measure the distance between the tip of the chin and the suprasternal notch (extension).
Trick movement: Mouth opening.

Neck extension using an inclinometer

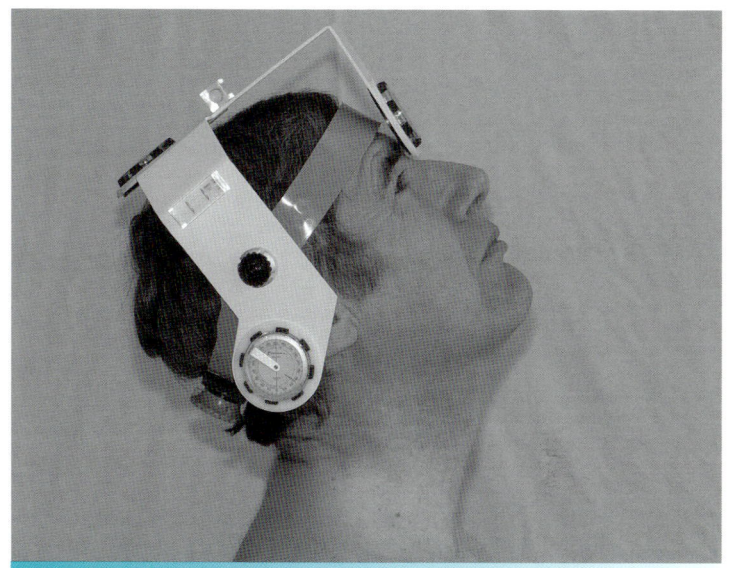

Fig 8.10 Measurement of neck extension using an inclinometer.

Starting position: The patient is positioned in sitting, head and neck in the anatomical position (see Fig. 8.7). Ensure that the measurement device is horizontal on the patient's head and the inclinometer should read zero.
Command to patient: 'Look up to the ceiling as far as you can.'
End position: The patient extends the neck to the limit of motion.

THE SPINE

Neck lateral flexion using a tape measure

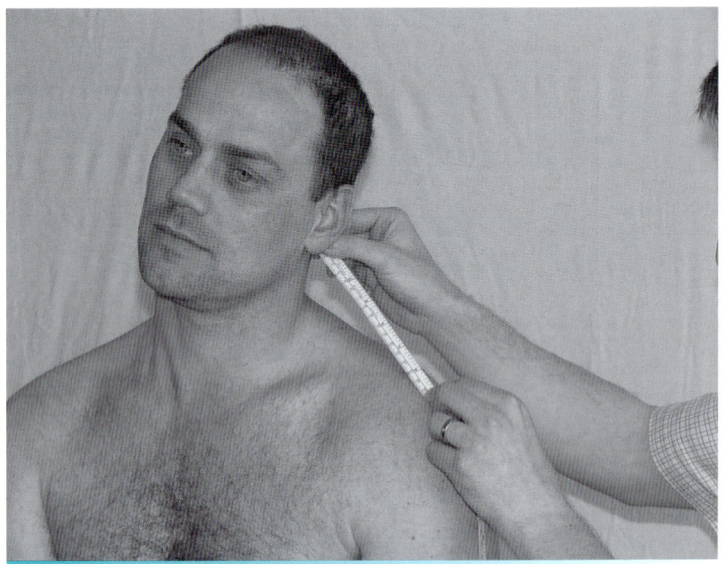

Fig 8.11 Measurement of neck lateral flexion (side flexion) using a tape measure.

Starting position: The patient is positioned in sitting, head and neck in the anatomical position.
Command to patient: 'Take your ear down to your shoulder as far as you can.'
End position: The patient flexes the neck to the side (lateral flexion), to the limit of motion.
Measurement: A tape measure measures the distance between the mastoid process and the acromion process (lateral flexion).
Trick movement: Elevation of the shoulder girdle towards the ear.

Measure the range of movement to the opposite side.

Neck lateral flexion using an inclinometer

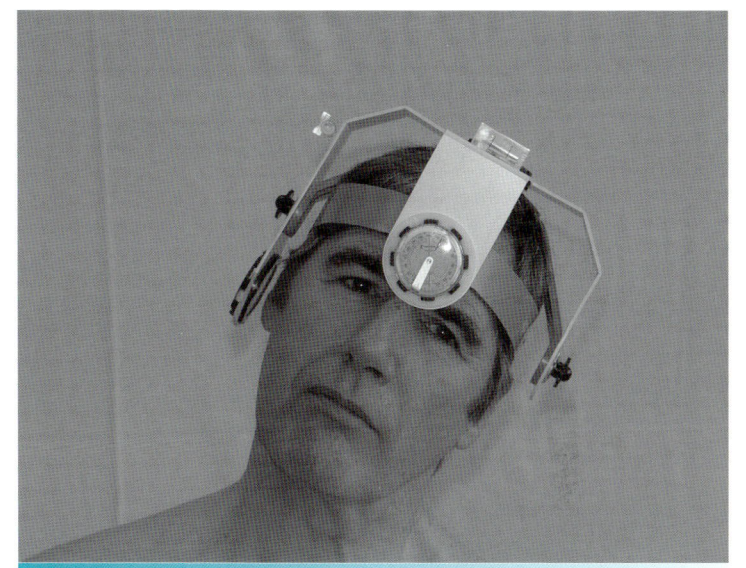

Fig 8.12 Measurement of neck lateral flexion using a cervical measurement system.

Starting position: The patient is positioned in sitting, head and neck in the anatomical position (see Fig. 8.7). Ensure that the measurement device is horizontal on the patient's head and the inclinometer should read zero.
Command to patient: 'Take your ear down to your shoulder as far as you can.'
End position: The patient flexes the neck to the side to the limit of motion.

Measure the range of movement to the opposite side.

Neck rotation using a tape measure

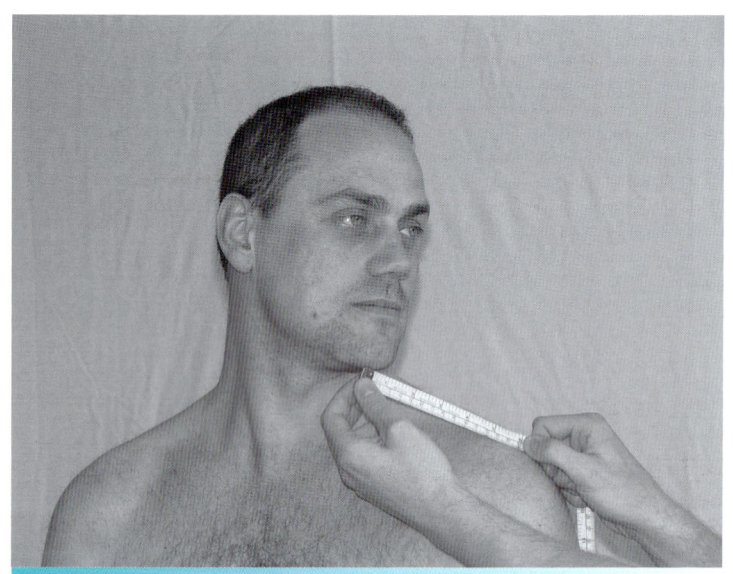

Fig 8.13 Measurement of neck rotation using a tape measure.

Starting position: The patient is positioned in sitting, head and neck in the anatomical position.
Command to patient: 'Turn your head round to your left (or right) shoulder as far as you can.'
End position: The patient rotates the head to the limit of motion.
Measurement: A tape is used to measure the distance between the tip of the chin and the acromion process (rotation).
Trick movement: Elevation and/or protraction of the shoulder girdle.

Measure the range of movement to the opposite side.

Measurement of neck rotation using a compass goniometer

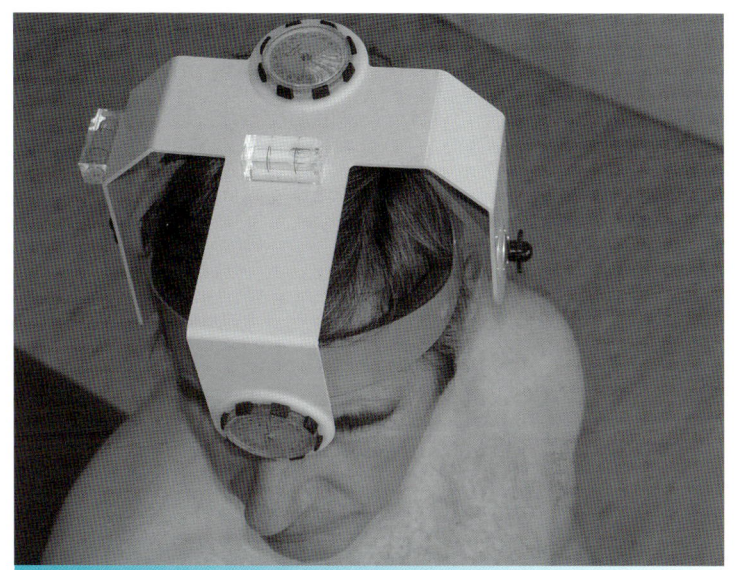

Fig 8.14 Measurement of neck rotation using a cervical measurement system.

Starting position: The patient is positioned in sitting, head and neck in the anatomical position (see Fig. 8.7). Ensure that the measurement device is horizontal on the patient's head and the compass goniometer should read zero.
Command to patient: 'Turn your head round to your left (or right) shoulder as far as you can.'
End position: The patient rotates the neck to the limit of motion.

Measure the range of movement to the opposite side.

THE SPINE

Notes

Treatment record

CHAPTER 9

The respiratory system

ANATOMY 209
  Bony landmarks to be palpated 209
  Muscles 210
  Joints of the thorax 210
    Sternal joints 210
    Sternocostal joints 211
    Ligaments 211
    Costochondral joint 211
    Interchondral joints 211
    Costotransverse joint 212
    Ligaments 212
    Costovertebral joint 212
    Ligaments 213
  Measurement 213
  Chest expansion 213
  Respiratory function 216
    FEV_1 and FVC 216
    Peak expiratory flow rate (PEFR) 218

ANATOMY

1. The bony components of the thorax articulate with one another in such a way as to provide a rigid, yet slightly mobile thoracic cage.
2. It is the articulation of the rib with the vertebral column posteriorly and with the sternum anteriorly, which provides the mobility necessary during respiration.
3. By the action of the muscles, the ribs are moved so as to change the anteroposterior and transverse diameters of the thorax.
4. The main muscles of respiration are the diaphragm and the intercostal muscles.

BONY LANDMARKS TO BE PALPATED

Spinous processes in the thoracic region, thoracic transverse processes, ribs, manubrium, sternum and xiphoid process.

MUSCLES

Table 9.1

The muscles of inspiration (diaphragm and intercostals)

Muscle	Origin	Insertion	Nerve supply	Action(s)
Diaphragm	The right and left crura, the medial and lateral arcuate ligaments, inner surfaces of the lower six ribs and costal cartilages, and xiphoid process	The central tendon	Left and right phrenic nerve C3, 4, 5	Major muscle of inspiration The lower ribs are lifted upwards and outwards. The upper ribs push the sternum forwards Will assist in venous and lymphatic drainage
Intercostals: External – intercostals Internal – intercostal Innermost – intercostals	Lower border of the rib above Costal groove of the rib above Runs between innermost surfaces of adjacent ribs	Upper border of the rib below Upper border of the rib below	Anterior primary rami of adjacent intercostal nerves	Elevation of the rib below to the rib above, inspiration It produces a rigid cavity upon which the diaphragm can act

JOINTS OF THE THORAX (from anterior to posterior)

Sternal joints

Manubriosternal joint:

1. This is a secondary cartilaginous joint.
2. It is an articulation between the inferior surface of the manubrium and the upper surface of the body of the sternum.
3. The opposing surfaces of the two bones are covered with a thin layer of hyaline cartilage, between which there is a fibrocartilaginous disc.
4. A small amount of movement (7°) is permitted at this joint. During inspiration there is a decrease in the obtuse angle between the manubrium and the body of the sternum.
5. The joint is strengthened in front and behind by longitudinal fibrous bands and the adjacent sternocostal (radiate) ligaments.

Xiphisternal joint
1. This is a secondary cartilaginous joint.
2. It is an articulation between the xiphoid process and the body of the sternum.
3. The xiphoid process is an irregularly shaped piece of cartilage.
4. It is supported all round by a fibrous capsule.
5. While it remains cartilaginous, there is a certain amount of flexibility of the xiphoid process at the joint.

Sternocostal joints
1. These are joints between the medial end of the costal cartilage of the 1st to 7th ribs and the sternum.
2. The joints between the 1st costal cartilage and the sternum is a primary cartilaginous joint.
3. The remaining joints are synovial.
4. They are surrounded by a fibrous capsule.

Ligaments
Table 9.4

Ligaments		
Ligaments	Origin	Insertion
The anterior radiate ligament	From the medial end of the costal cartilage	Three bands insert into the anterior aspect of the sternum, passing upwards, horizontally and inferiorly
The posterior radiate ligament	From the medial end of the costal cartilage	Three bands insert into the posterior aspect of the sternum, passing upwards, horizontally

Costochondral joint
1. This is a primary cartilaginous joint.
2. It is an articulation between the anterior roughened end of a rib and the lateral end of the costal cartilage.
3. It is surrounded by perichondrium, which is continuous with the periosteum of the rib.
4. Movement at these joints is confined to a slight bending of the cartilage at the junction of the rib.
5. The cartilage may, however, show some twisting movement of the sternum.

Interchondral joints
1. These joints are between the tips of the costal cartilages of the 8th, 9th and 10th ribs and the lower border of the cartilage above.

2. The 8th and 9th joints are synovial, whereas the 10th is a fibrous joint.
3. The joints are surrounded by a fibrous capsule.
4. They are strengthened anteriorly and posteriorly by oblique ligaments.
5. The joints provide a slight gliding movement.

Costotransverse joint

1. The costotransverse joint is a synovial joint.
2. It is an articulation between articular facet on the transverse process of the vertebra near its tip and an oval facet on the posteromedial aspect of the tubercle of the rib.
3. A thin, fibrous capsule completely surrounds the joint.
4. In the lower joints there is gliding and rotation of one plane surface against another.
5. In the higher joints, because of the curved joint surfaces, there is rotation.

Ligaments

Table 9.2

Ligaments		
Ligament	Origin	Insertion
Lateral costotransverse ligament	The tip of the transverse process	The roughened lateral part of the costal tubercle
Costotransverse ligament	The back of the neck of the rib	To the front of the transverse process
Superior costotransverse ligament	The rib – an anterior and posterior band	The undersurface of the transverse process of the vertebra above

Costovertebral joint

1. This is a synovial joint.
2. It is an articulation between articular facets on the head of the rib and the demi-facet on the upper border of the corresponding vertebra and a smaller demi-facet on the lower border of the vertebra above.
3. The crest of the head of the rib articulates with a slight depression on the posterolateral aspect of the intervening intervertebral disc.
4. An intra-articular ligament completely divides the joint space.
5. A loose, fibrous capsule surrounds the joint.

Ligaments

Table 9.3

Ligaments		
Ligament	**Origin**	**Insertion**
Radiate ligament of the head of the rib	From the front of the head of the rib	Three bands – to the body of the vertebra above, horizontally to the intervertebral disc, inferiorly to the body of the vertebra below

MEASUREMENT

CHEST EXPANSION

Starting position: The patient is positioned in a safe sitting position or standing, arms at their side.

Equipment: Flexible tape measure and surface marking pen.

Apical measurement

1. Place the tape around the chest wall in line with the axilla. Ensure that tape is not twisted and is in parallel both anteriorly and posteriorly.
2. Place a visible mark on the model to indicate the tape position.

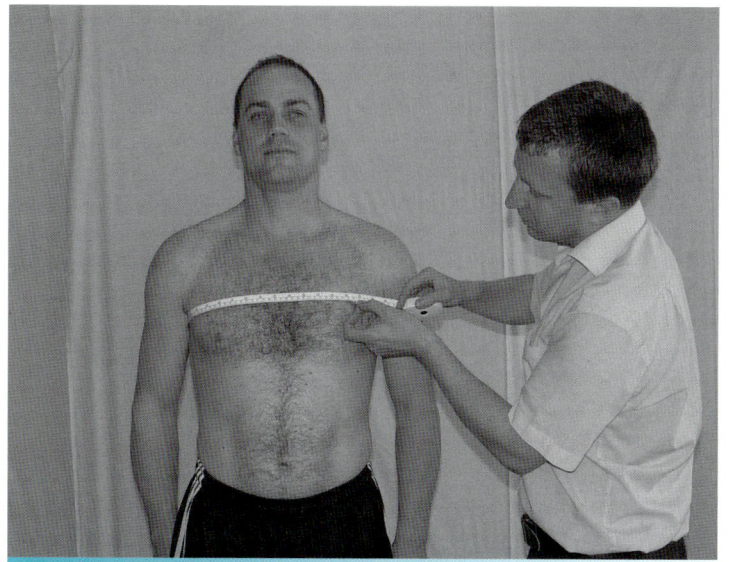

Fig 9.1 Measurement of apical chest expansion using a tape measure.

3. Take a measurement on full *expiration*.
4. Holding the tape in position, ask the patient to breathe in as much as they can, to full inspiration.
5. Take the measurement at full *inspiration*.
6. Calculate the difference.
7. Using your mark as a guide, repeat stages 3–5 twice, until you have three measurements of expiration and inspiration.

Basal measurement 1

1. Place the tape around the chest wall in line with the xiphoid process of the sternum. Ensure that the tape is not twisted and is in parallel both anteriorly and posteriorly.
2. Place a visible mark on the model to indicate the tape position.
3. Take a measurement on *expiration*.
4. Holding the tape in position, ask the patient to breathe in as much as they can, to full inspiration.
5. Take a measurement at full *inspiration*.
6. Calculate the difference.
7. Using your mark as a guide, repeat stages 3–5 twice, until you have three measurements of expiration and inspiration.

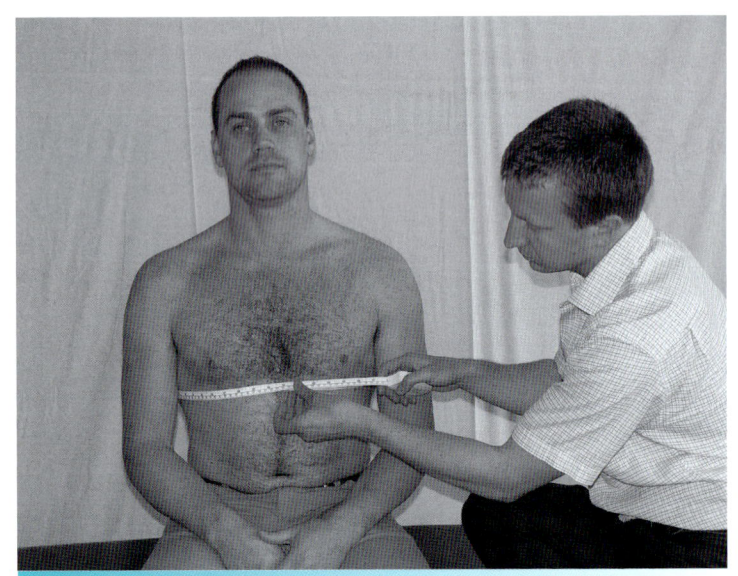

Fig 9.2 Measurement of basal chest expansion using a tape measure.

Basal measurement 2

1. Place the tape around the chest wall in line with the xiphoid process of the sternum. Ensure that the tape is not twisted and is in parallel both anteriorly and posteriorly.
2. Place a visible mark on the model to indicate the tape position.
3. Take a measurement on *expiration*.
4. Holding the tape in position, ask the patient to breathe in as much as they can, to full inspiration.
5. Take a measurement at full *inspiration*.
6. Calculate the difference.
7. Using your mark as a guide, repeat stages 3–5 twice, until you have three measurements of expiration and inspiration.

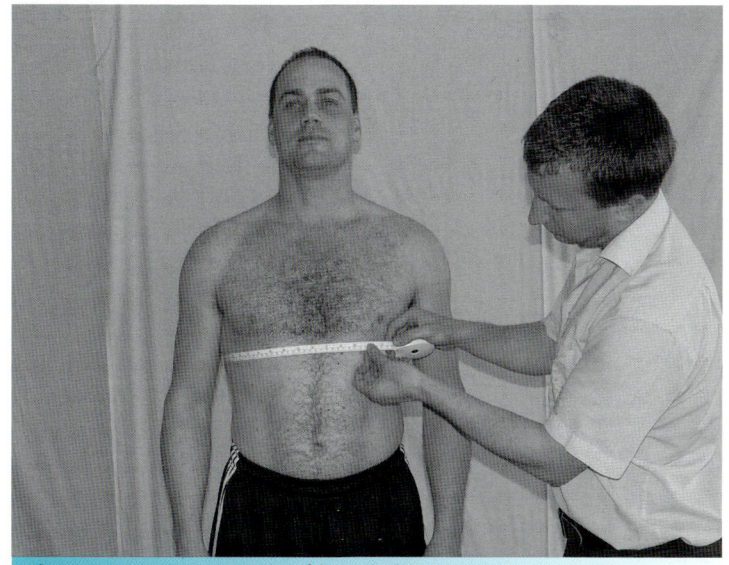

Fig 9.3 Measurement of basal chest expansion using a tape measure.

RESPIRATORY FUNCTION
FEV_1 and FVC (AARC 1996)
(Forced expiratory volume in 1 second and Forced vital capacity)

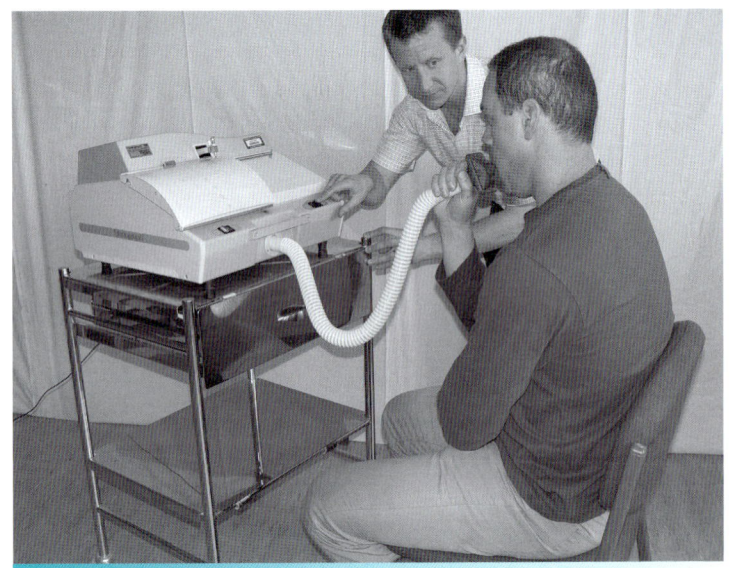

Fig 9.4 Measurement of FEV_1 and FVC using a Vitalograph.

Equipment
- Mouthpiece
- Filter
- Spirometer
- Nose clip (optional)

Patient preparation: Obtain the height and weight of the patient. Always check for contraindications. Explain the purpose and nature of the test to the patient. Place the patient in a safe, comfortable sitting position, close to the spirometer.

Instructions: Ensure that a new mouthpiece and filter are fitted to the tube of the spirometer (Vitalograph). This is important to avoid any cross-infection.

The Vitalogram chart is placed correctly (upside down) in the chart carrier. The stylus is placed on the stylus start position, marked on the top right-hand corner of the chart.

Instruct the patient to breathe as deeply as possible (to full inspiration), to place the lips tightly around the mouthpiece and then to blow out into the mouthpiece as hard and fast as possible, until no further gas can be exhaled.

As soon as the patient commences to blow into the mouthpiece, the machine is set to record by the clinician pressing the record switch. The stylus then draws a mark on the chart, as the carrier moves from left to right.

The patient should continue blowing out until a full recording has taken place. The patient should be encouraged to keep blowing for the full 6/7 seconds of the test. The patient should prevent their tongue from occluding the mouthpiece and their teeth should be placed around the outside of the mouthpiece, if it is a rigid tube.

The operator should observe the patient at all times to confirm a reliable technique.

Three trials are performed. The clinician then calculates the FEV_1 and FVC from the patient's chart.

Contraindications: Haemoptysis, pneumothorax, unstable cardiovascular status, aneurysms, recent eye surgery, acute illness, recent surgery to thorax or abdomen, pregnancy.

REFERENCE

AARC 1996 Clinical practice guidelines. Respiratory Care 41: 629–636

Peak expiratory flow rate (PEFR)

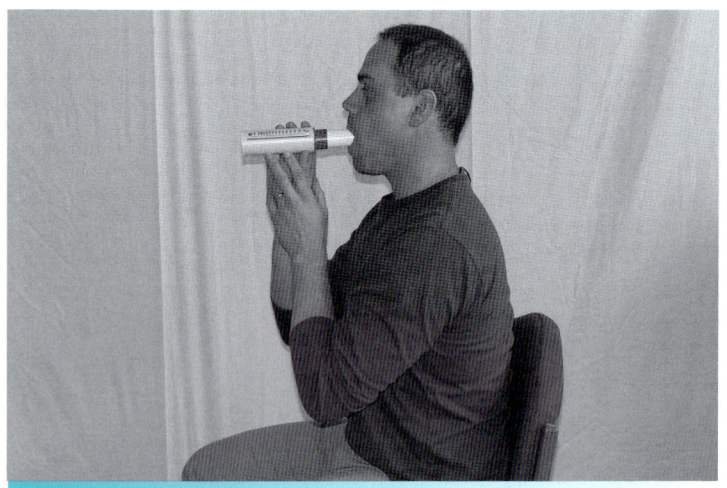

Fig 9.5 Measurement of peak expiratory flow rate (PEFR) using a peak flow meter.

Equipment
- Peak flow meter (single patient use)
- Mouthpiece
- Filter (if required)

Patient preparation: Explain the purpose and nature of the test to the patient. Place the patient in a safe, comfortable sitting position.
Instructions: If the patient is using hospital equipment, then a new mouthpiece and filter should be fitted to the peak flow meter. This is to avoid any cross-infection.

Instruct the patient to breathe as deeply as possible (to full inspiration), and to place their lips tightly around the mouthpiece, to ensure a good seal. The teeth should be placed around the outside of the mouthpiece, if it is a rigid tube, and the patient should prevent the tongue from occluding the mouthpiece. The patient then makes a short, sharp, hard blow into the peak flow meter with an open glottis. The blow can be stopped after about 1 second. The operator should observe the patient at all times to confirm a reliable technique.

The highest reading of at least three acceptable blows should be recorded, with the pointer being returned to zero between each blow.

APPENDIX 1

The visual analogue scale for pain

The visual analogue scale (VAS) is a tool widely used in medical practice to measure pain. It has been used clinically since the late 1970s and, along with the numeric rating scale (NRS), is still one of the main measures of pain outcomes in physiotherapy.

The VAS is a simple measuring tool, where the patient indicates, by making a mark along a 10 cm horizontal or vertical line, their perceived pain intensity at that moment in time. The left-hand border, A, represents no pain and the right-hand border, B, represents the worse pain imaginable. The clinician measures from the left-hand border, A, to the mark the patient has made on the line. This then will be their VAS score. As the patient's pain reduces, their VAS score will also reduce.

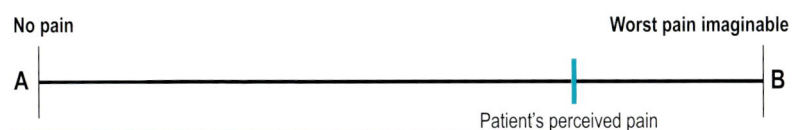

Figure A.1 The 10 cm visual analogue scale (VAS).

The Numeric Rating Scale (NRS)

This is another tool used for measuring pain. The patient is asked to rate their pain at that moment in time, using numbers, usually 0–10 (11 points) or 0–20 (21 points). The anchor points are at the 0 point "no pain" and the 10 or 20 point "worst pain possible".

FURTHER READING

Lundeberg T, Lund I, Dahlin L et al 2001 Reliability and responsiveness of three different pain assessments. Journal of Rehabilitation and Medicine 33:279–283

Litcher-Kelly L, Martino SA, Broderick JE, Stone AA 2007 A systematic review of measures used to assess chronic musculoskeletal pain in the clinical and randomized controlled clinical trials. Journal of Pain 8(12):906–913

APPENDIX 2

Summary of studies assessing the reliability and validity of measuring tools in physiotherapy

Studies assessing reliability and validity

Table A.1

Goniometer

Study	Aim of study	Numbers	Methodology	Results
Armstrong et al (1998)	To examine the intratester, intertester and inter-device reliability of range of motion measurements of the elbow and forearm. For the inter-device reliability the authors compared a universal goniometer with a computerized goniometer and a mechanical rotation measuring device	38 subjects, who had undergone a surgical procedure for an injury to the elbow, forearm or wrist participated in the study. Five testers measured each subject	Elbow flexion and extension, pronation and supination were measured using a standardized test method and a randomized order of testing	The intraclass correlation coefficients (ICCs) for intratester reliability were high for active elbow flexion and extension and pronation and supination with all three instruments, with 57 of 60 ICCs exceeding 0.89. The ICCs for intertester reliability for elbow flexion and extension measurements were moderate for the universal goniometer and high for the computerized goniometer. For supination and pronation all three instruments showed high intraclass correlation coefficients. The authors conclude that measurement error is small when the same tester repeats a measure with the same device
Bierma-Zeinstra et al (1998)	To compare the reliability of measurements of hip motions obtained with an electronic inclinometer and a two-arm goniometer	Nine healthy subjects participated in the study. 10 medically educated observers performed the hip measurements with the two instruments	To examine the intraobserver variability, one observer measured the various hip movements 10 times consecutively in the nine subjects, using both instruments	The two instruments showed equal intraobserver variability for the hip movements in general. The authors conclude that the electronic inclinometer is more reliable in measurements of hip rotation, but for hip movements in general the two-arm goniometer is just as accurate when used by one observer

(table continues)

Table A.1 (continued)

Study	Aim of study	Numbers	Methodology	Results
			To examine the interobserver variability 10 different observers measured the hip movements of the nine subjects, using the two instruments	
Brosseau et al (2001)	To study the intratester and intertester reliability of the universal goniometer (UG) and the parallelogram goniometer (PG) for active knee flexion and extension on subjects with knee restrictions To examine the criterion validity of both goniometers To examine the criterion validity of visual estimations	60 subjects with a knee impairment participated in the study	The first tester visually estimated the active range of motion (AROM) of knee flexion and extension. They then measured the AROM of flexion and extension with the UG and PG. A radiograph of the knee joint movements was also obtained. A recorder collated the measurements The second tester then performed the same measurements. These were again collated by a recorder Both testers then performed the same measurements a second time	The UG intratester reliability of measurements for flexion, using the intraclass correlation coefficients (ICCs), was 0.997 and for extension was 0.972 to 0.985 The PG intratester reliability of measurements for flexion, using the ICCs, was 0.996 and for extension 0.953 to 0.955 The UG intertester reliability of measurements for flexion, using the ICCs, was 0.926 to 0.977 and for extension 0.893 to 0.926 The PG intertester reliability of measurements for flexion, using the ICCs, was 0.959 to 0.970 and for extension 0.856 to 0.898

Croxford et al (1998)	To examine the intertester variability, measurement error and concurrent validity of measurements of active ankle dorsiflexion using the universal goniometer (UG) and visual estimation (VE)	12 experienced physiotherapists were randomly selected to participate in the study	Each of the 12 participants measured the full range of ankle dorsiflexion of a healthy subject. They first assessed dorsiflexion of the ankle joint visually and then measured dorsiflexion using a masked universal goniometer. This was read and documented by a recorder	The results showed that intertester variation of visual estimation was twice as great as that obtained using the goniometer (coefficient of variation for VE was 69% and for UG was 35%) The measurement error was 111° for VE and 55° for UG The testers in the study did not use a standardized measuring protocol The authors conclude that therapists should use a goniometer to measure joint range of movement and a standardized measuring protocol
Gajdosik & Bohannon (1987)	The purpose of the article is to review the literature on the reliability and validity of goniometric measurements of the extremities		The authors define reliability and review the literature, discussing instrumentation and measuring procedures, passive versus active measurements, intratester versus intertester measurements and validity in goniometric measurement	The authors conclude that therapists should adopt standardized methods of testing and should interpret and report goniometric results as range of motion measurements only

(table continues)

Table A.1 (continued)

Study	Aim of study	Numbers	Methodology	Results
Holm et al (2000)	To study the reliability of goniometric measurements and visual estimates of hip range of movement (ROM) in patients with osteoarthrosis (OA)	25 patients with OA hip participated in the study and had all hip movements measured on two occasions	Five testers, full-time physiotherapists, were divided into three measuring teams. They measured all hip movements (flexion, extension, abduction, adduction, internal and external rotation) on two occasions with a goniometer. An orthopaedic surgeon made visual assessments of the hip movements	There were no significant differences between measurements recorded on the first and second occasions for the same team There was a high agreement between goniometric measurement and visual estimation
Jordan (2000)	To assess the reliability of tools to measure cervical spine range of motion (ROM) in clinical settings		This paper is a systematic review of the tools to measure ROM of the cervical spine. The author reviews 21 papers, which are presented in table form	
LaStayo & Wheeler (1994)	To determine whether passive wrist flexion and extension goniometric measurements using ulnar alignment, radial alignment and volar/dorsal alignment were similar or dissimilar	140 patients (141 wrists) participated in the study and were tested by 32 therapists in eight clinics around the USA. At each clinic, measurements	The first tester measured the passive wrist extension and flexion of the subject with a 152 cm masked goniometer. A recorder read and documented each measurement	The intratester reliability of measurements for flexion, using the intraclass correlation coefficients (ICCs) for the radial, ulnar and dorsal alignment techniques, were 0.86, 0.87 and 0.92, respectively The intratester reliability of measurements for extension, using the ICCs for the radial,

	To examine which of the three techniques had the greatest intratester and intertester reliability	of subjects were performed by randomly paired sets of testers	After an interval of 30–60 seconds the tester re-measured the subject After an interval of 2–3 minutes a second tester repeated all the measurements twice while the recorder documented the results	ulnar and dorsal alignment techniques, were 0.80, 0.80, and 0.84, respectively Intertester reliability of measurements for flexion, using the ICC for the radial, ulnar and dorsal alignment techniques, were 0.88, 0.89 and 0.93, respectively Intertester reliability of measurements for extension, using the ICC for the radial, ulnar and dorsal alignment techniques, were 0.80, 0.80 and 0.84 respectively The authors conclude that the overall results indicated there were differences among the three goniometric techniques
Sabari et al (1998)	To examine the difference in goniometric measurements of active range of motion (AROM) and passive range of motion (PROM) of shoulder flexion and abduction when movements were assessed in the sitting, as compared to the supine position	30 adults (age range 17–92) participated in the study	Each subject was measured eight times: AROM and PROM for shoulder flexion and abduction were measured with the patient in both sitting position and supine position. The tester aligned the goniometer and an assistant read and recorded the data	Intraclass correlation coefficients (ICCs) ranged from 0.94 to 0.99, indicating extremely high intrarater reliability when measuring AROM and PROM of shoulder flexion and abduction in the supine or sitting position

(table continues)

Table A.1 (continued)

Study	Aim of study	Numbers	Methodology	Results
Watkins et al (1991)	To examine the intratester and intertester reliability of goniometric measurements of knee flexion and extension passive range of motion (PROM) To examine the parallel-forms intratester reliability for goniometric measurements and visual estimates for knee flexion and extension To examine the parallel-forms intertester reliability for goniometric measurements and visual estimates for knee flexion and extension To examine intertester reliability for visual estimates of knee flexion and extension	43 patients (50 knees) received repeated measures in a clinical setting. 14 therapists performed the measurements	The first tester visually estimated the PROM of knee flexion and extension. The results were documented by the recorder They then measured twice the passive knee flexion and extension of the subject with a 12.7 cm masked goniometer. The recorder read the values and documented them A second tester took the same six measurements in the same order. These were also documented by the recorder	The intraclass correlation coefficients (ICCs) for intratester reliability of measurements obtained with a goniometer were 0.99 for knee flexion and 0.98 for knee extension The ICC values for intertester reliability of measurements obtained with a goniometer were 0.90 for knee flexion and 0.86 for knee extension The ICC values for the parallel-forms intratester reliability of goniometric measurements and visual estimates were 0.93 for flexion and 0.94 for extension The ICC values for the parallel-forms intertester reliability of goniometric measurements and visual estimates were 0.86 for flexion and 0.82 for extension The ICC values for intertester reliability of visual estimates were 0.83 for flexion and 0.82 for extension
Williams & Callaghan (1990)	To compare the performance of practised and non-practised groups of physiotherapists in the assessment of a joint angle using visual estimation and three different types of goniometer	22 chartered physiotherapists were divided into two groups – those who measured daily and those who measured infrequently	Each group of physiotherapists visually assessed the range of shoulder flexion of a subject (100°) and then measured once the range of shoulder flexion using the three types of	The practised group had a mean visual estimation of 106.36°, and goniometric measurements of (i) 102.27°, (ii) 101.36° and (iii) 104.27° The non-practised group had a mean visual estimation of 103.36°, and goniometric measurements of (i) 105° (ii) 101.81° and (iii) 102.63°

Youdas et al (1993)	To evaluate the degree of intratester reliability for active range of motion (AROM) measurements of ankle dorsiflexion (ADF) and ankle plantarflexion (APF) obtained with the universal goniometer (UG) To evaluate the degree of intertester reliability for AROM measurements of ADF and APF obtained using visual estimation (VE) and universal goniometer (UG) To evaluate the degree of parallel-forms intratester reliability when repeated measurements are made on the same subject by the same tester using VE and UG	45 ankles were measured using 38 patients with primary ankle complaints	10 physical therapists performed the measurements using VE and the UG Each therapist measured nine different patients and was paired with each of the other nine clinicians The first therapist visually estimated and recorded the AROM of ADF and APF. They then used the masked UG and measured AROM of ADF twice and APF twice. The clinician was permitted to use their own measuring protocol. The second therapist then performed the six measurements in the same sequence. All the readings were collated by a recorder	The authors conclude that for highly skilled clinicians, visual estimation is the more valid technique and goniometers may be redundant The intratester reliability of measurements obtained with the UG using the intraclass correlation coefficients (ICC) for ADF were 0.64 to 0.92 and for APF were 0.47 to 0.96 Intertester reliability of measurements obtained with the UG using the ICC for ADF were 0.28 and for APF were 0.25 The ICC for VE for ADF was 0.34 and for APF was 0.48 The ICC for parallel-forms intratester reliability obtained with the UG and VE for ADF ranged from 0 to 0.94 and for APF ranged from 0 to 0.86 The authors conclude that a therapist should use a goniometer when repeatedly measuring AROM of the ankle joint
Youdas et al (1992)	To determine normal values of cervical active range of	337 healthy volunteers (171 females and		The median intraclass correlation coefficients (ICCs) demonstrated that

(table continues)

Table A.1 (continued)

Study	Aim of study	Numbers	Methodology	Results
	motion (AROM) by using the cervical range of motion (CROM) instrument on a large number of healthy volunteers whose ages spanned nine decades	166 males) ranging in age from 11 to 97 participated in the study	measurements of cervical AROM with the CROM, each of the five testers made repeated AROM measurements on six healthy subjects	intratester reliability was fair for neck flexion (ICC = 0.76); high for neck extension (ICC = 0.94); and good for neck left lateral flexion (ICC = 0.86), right lateral flexion (ICC = 0.85), left rotation (ICC = 0.84) and right rotation (ICC = 0.80)
	To determine whether age and gender affect the six cervical movements	Generally, there were 40 subjects in each group, except in the 90–97-year-old group, which contained 14 subjects	Each subject performed three repetitions of neck flexion, extension, left and right lateral flexion and left and right rotation	Intertester reliability was high for neck extension (ICC = 0.90) and good for neck extension (ICC = 0.83), left and right lateral flexion (ICC = 0.89 and 0.87, respectively) and right rotation (ICC = 0.82). Left rotation showed poor reliability (ICC = 0.66)
	To examine the intratester and intertester reliability of measurements of cervical AROM with the CROM device	The measurements were taken by five physical therapists	The subjects repeated the same movements, providing two sets of six measurements	The authors conclude that with each 10-year change in age, they believe that both sexes will lose approximately five degrees of neck extension AROM and three degrees of AROM for each of the four other neck movements
			To investigate the intertester reliability of measurements of cervical AROM with the CROM, 20 different healthy volunteers participated	
			Each subject's six cervical AROM movements were measured independently by three testers using the same device within minutes of each other	

REFERENCES

Armstrong AD, MacDermid JC, Chinchalker S, Stevens RS, King GJW 1998 Reliability of range-of-motion in the elbow and forearm. Journal of Shoulder and Elbow Surgery 7(6):573–580

Bierma-Zeinstra SMA, Bohnen AM, Ramial R et al 1998 Comparison between two devices for measuring hip joint motion. Clinical Rehabilitation 12(6):497–505

Brosseau L, Balmer S, Tousignant M et al 2001 Intra- and inter-tester reliability and criterion validity of the parallelogram of universal goniometers for measuring maximum active knee flexion and extension of patients with knee restriction. Archives of Physical and Medical Rehabilitation 82(3):396–402

Croxford P, Jones K, Barker K 1998 Inter-tester comparison between visual estimation and goniometric measurement of ankle dorsiflexion. Physiotherapy Theory and Practice 14(2):107–113

Gajdosik RL, Bohannon RW 1987 Clinical measurement of range of motion: review of goniometry emphasizing reliability and validity. Physical Therapy 67(12):1867–1872

Holm I, Bolstad B, Lütken T et al 2000 Reliability of goniometric measurements and visual estimates of hip ROM in patients with osteoarthrosis. Physiotherapy Research International 5(4):241–248

Jordan K 2000 Assessment of published reliability studies for cervical spine range-of-motion measurement tools. Journal of Manipulative and Physiological Therapeutics 23(3):180–195

LaStayo PC, Wheeler DL 1994 Reliability of passive wrist flexion and extension goniometric measurements: a multicenter study. Physical Therapy 74(2):162–176

Sabari JS, Maltzev I, Lubarsky D et al 1998 Goniometric assessment of shoulder range of motion: comparison of testing in supine and sitting positions. Archives of Physical Medicine and Rehabilitation 79(6):647–651

Watkins MA, Riddle DL, Lamb RL et al 1991 Reliability of goniometric measurements and visual estimates of knee range of motion obtained in a clinical setting. Physical Therapy 71(2):90–98

Williams JG, Callaghan M 1990 Comparison of visual estimation and goniometry in determination of a shoulder joint angle. Physiotherapy 76(10):655–657

Youdas JW, Bogard CL, Suman VJ 1993 Reliability of goniometric measurements and visual estimates of ankle joint active range of motion obtained in a clinical setting. Archives of Physical Medicine and Rehabilitation 74(10):1113–1118

Youdas JW, Garrett TR, Suman VJ, Bogard CL, Hallman HO, Carey JR 1992 Normal range of motion of the cervical spine: an initial goniometric study. Physical Therapy 72(11):770–780

Table A.2

Tape measure: limb/joint girth

Study	Aim of study	Numbers	Methodology	Results
Karges et al (2003)	To determine the concurrent validity of the calculated volume derived from circumference measurements and water displacement volume in oedematous (lymphoedematous) and non-oedematous upper extremities	A convenience sample of 14 women with a diagnosis of upper extremity lymphoedema participated in the study	The participants were instructed on how to appropriately place their upper limb in the volumeter. The overflow from the volumeter was collected and the amount of water was recorded as the upper extremity water displacement volume of the limb. A second volumetric test was undertaken, where the hand was lowered into the water to the level of the finger MCP joints. The overflow was recorded as the finger volume. The upper extremity to finger water displacement was determined by subtracting the finger volume from the upper extremity volume. Circumference measurements were taken on the upper extremity using a standard tape measure. Measurements were taken at the following points: finger MCP joints, thumb MCP joint, wrist, and proximal from the wrist in 4cm increments and the elbow. The most proximal measurement point was between the mid-humerus and axilla. From these measurements the data were entered into a computer and the volume was calculated, based on the frustrum formula	The intraclass correlation coefficient (ICC) for calculated volume (circumference measurements) versus water displacement volume was 0.99. The authors conclude that the reliability of the calculated volume measurements was comparable to the reliability of the water displacement volume measurements. The calculated volume and water displacement volume measures were highly associated, whether looking at volume or side-to-side differences

Labs et al (2000)	To compare the reliability of repeated spring tape measurements with optoelectronic volumeter measurements for the assessment of lower leg circumferences	30 healthy volunteers participated in the study	The subjects were positioned in half sitting with their lower leg in hip and knee flexion, their foot resting on a foot rest The limb circumference at mid-calf and ankle level of both legs was measured three times using a spring tape measure and an optoelectronic volumeter. The entire procedure was repeated on the other leg	The circumference measures taken by a spring tape measure and optoelectronic volumetry are both highly reliable methods
Soderberg et al (1996)	To determine the intra- and interrater reliability of lower extremity girth measurements in patients recovering from anterior cruciate ligament (ACL) reconstructive surgery	Nine subjects, within several months of their surgery, participated in the study Three physical therapists performed the measurements	The subjects were positioned in supine lying, with their knee in full extension Both lower limb girths were measured, using the following locations: 15 cm inferior to the knee joint line; at the joint line; at 5 cm, 10 cm and 15 cm above the joint line and at mid-thigh The three clinicians measured the limb girth at the six locations on both legs on two occasions on the same day	The intratester intraclass coefficient (ICCs) showed high coefficients (0.82–1.0) for both the involved and uninvolved legs for all the locations of the measurement Intertester ICCs ranged from 0.72 to 0.97 The authors conclude that the circumferential measurements of subjects with ACL-deficient knees, who are recovering from surgery, can be reliably measured by physical therapists

(table continues)

STUDIES ASSESSING RELIABILITY AND VALIDITY

Table A.2 (continued)

Study	Aim of study	Numbers	Methodology	Results
Taylor et al (2006)	To assess the reliability and validity of circumferential measurements and water displacement for measuring upper-limb volume	66 female subjects participated in the study and were divided into three groups. Two raters measured each subject	Group 1: (25 subjects) were in a control group. Group 2: (22 subjects) were in the breast cancer group, without a diagnosis of arm lymphoedema. Group 3: (19 subjects) were diagnosed with arm lymphoedema, following breast cancer surgery. Two raters measured each subject by using circumferential tape measurements at specific distances from the fingertips and in relation to anatomical landmarks and by using water displacement	The interrater reliability values based on the two raters were 0.98–0.99 for the circumferential tape measurements at 30–60 cm from the fingertips. The interrater reliability values for the five circumferential measurements taken in relation to the three bony landmarks (wrist at styloid, elbow at olecranon and shoulder at acromion) were 0.97–0.99. The authors conclude that the study has shown that arm circumferential measurements in relation to anatomic landmarks are reliable and valid measurements of arm volumes

REFERENCES

Karges JR, Mark BE, Stikeleather SJ, Worrell TW 2003 Concurrent validity of upper-extremity volume estimates: comparison of calculated volume derived from girth measurements and water displacement volume. Physical Therapy 83(2):134–145

Labs KH, Tschoepl M, Gamba G et al 2000 The reliability of leg circumference assessment: a comparison of spring tape measurements and optoelectronic volumetry. Vascular Medicine 5(2):69–74

Soderberg GL, Ballantyne BT, Kestel LL 1996 Reliability of lower extremity girth measurements after anterior cruciate ligament reconstruction. Physiotherapy Research International 1(1):7–16

Taylor R, Jayasinghe UW, Keolmeyer L et al 2006 Reliability and validity of arm volume measurements for assessment of lymphoedema. Physical Therapy 86(2):205–214

Table A.3

Tape measure: leg length

Study	Aim of study	Numbers	Methodology	Results
Beattie et al (1990)	To determine the validity of leg length difference (LLD) measurements obtained with the tape measure method (TTM) as compared with LLD measurements obtained radiographically	10 subjects (patient group) with a history of LLD and nine healthy subjects (normal group) with no history of LLD participated in the study All the TTM measurements were taken by one examiner	The patient was positioned in supine lying, on the plinth. The examiner measured the leg length from the anterior superior iliac spine (ASIS) to the medial malleolus. The reading was recorded by another examiner. The procedure was repeated on the subject's opposite limb The subject was then asked to stand and move around for 1 minute. They were then positioned exactly as previously and the same examiner repeated the entire procedure, obtaining a second pair of measurements Every patient had radiographic measurements of leg length taken, with the technique based on the use of the mini-scanogram The intraclass correlation coefficient (ICC) was used to examine the degree of agreement for measurements taken in the study	The intraclass correlation coefficient (ICC) values obtained by comparing the first measurement of LLD obtained by the TTM with the measurement of LLD obtained using the mini-scanogram were 0.770 for the patient group, 0.359 for the normal group, and 0.683 for the entire sample The ICC values obtained by comparing the mean values of the two measurements of LLD obtained by the TTM with the measurement of LLD obtained using the mini-scanogram were 0.852 for the patient group, 0.637 for the normal group, and 0.793 for the entire sample The authors conclude that the measurements obtained with the TTM appear to be valid for assessing LLDs in patients when the mean of two measurements is used

Brady et al (2003)	To review the relevant literature concerning limb length inequalities in adults and to make recommendations for assessment and intervention based on the literature and their own clinical experience		The paper discusses the classification of limb length inequality, aetiological factors, pathologies related to limb length inequality and the assessment of limb length inequality. The sections on the clinical assessment of limb length inequality and the efficacy of lift intervention are particularly useful	The authors conclude that little agreement exists concerning the most accurate and useful method for detection of limb length inequality. If the tape measure method is used, measurement from the anterior superior iliac spine (ASIS) to the lateral malleolus is the most reliable technique, and using the mean of two measurements increases reliability
Gurney (2002)	To give an overview of the classification and aetiology of leg length discrepancy (LLD), the controversy of several measurement and treatment protocols, and a consolidation of research addressing the role of LLD on standing posture, standing balance, gait, running and various pathological conditions			
Harris et al (2005)	To assess the correlation between two commonly performed techniques of calculating leg length discrepancy (LLD): clinical	35 mature patients who had sustained a femoral shaft fracture	Leg length was measured with a tape measure using the anterior iliac spine and medial malleolus as reference points. A block test was also performed, where the patient was	There was a positive correlation between the leg length measurement with a tape measure and the block test ($P = 0.003$) There was no correlation between CT scanogram and the clinical measurement

(table continues)

Table A.3 (continued)

Study	Aim of study	Numbers	Methodology	Results
	examination and computed tomography (CT) scanogram	participated in the study	asked to stand with an adjustable raise under the short leg until it was felt the leg length was correct (using patient perception and pelvic obliquity) The block height was then measured in increments of 1 mm 29 of the patients had a CT scanogram performed The results of the clinical examination and scanogram were analysed using the Pearson product moment correlation	of leg length with the tape measure and the block test The authors conclude that their study has shown that physical examination (tape measure and block test) is more reliable and clinically relevant than CT scanogram measurement in the assessment of LLD after femoral fracture
Mannello (1992)	To review the literature pertaining to leg length inequality (LLI)		This paper discusses the classification of LLI, the incidence of LLI, the effects of asymmetry and methods of measurement or assessment of LLI. There is a useful section on orthopaedic procedures and measurement devices, which discusses the measurement of LLI using tape measure measurements and the block method	The author says that few definite conclusions can be made regarding the clinical orthopaedic methods for measuring LLI and more research is required before these methods are considered reliable and valid

| Middleton-Duff et al (2000) | To determine the criterion validity and intra- and intertester reliability of the tape and block methods of estimating leg length discrepancy (LLD) | 25 subjects participated in the study. 13 subjects were patients who had symptoms associated with LLD. 12 subjects were staff members, with no LLD problems

All the subjects were assessed by four podiatrists | For the tape measure method: all the subjects were lying supine on a plinth

Measurements of both legs were taken from the anterior superior iliac spine (ASIS) to the medial malleolus. The distance measured was read by an independent recorder

For the block method: all the subjects were standing with feet placed hip-width apart. Visual estimation was made of any asymmetry in the height of the left and right iliac crests. The tester placed a range of blocks under the foot of the lower side, until they believed the iliac crests to be level. The cumulative size of the blocks used was recorded

10 subjects had an X-ray performed | The intratester reliability for the block method was perfect

The tape method did produce some degree of intratester variability for all testers

The authors suggest that whilst the intratester reliability for the block method is better than the tape method, both approaches may be sensitive enough to differentiate 'large' clinically significant leg length discrepancy. They also suggest that the same tester should perform the assessment |

REFERENCES

Beattie P, Isaacson K, Riddle DL, Rothstein JM 1990 Validity of derived measurements of leg-length differences obtained by use of a tape measure. Physical Therapy 70(3):150–157

Brady RJ, Dean JB, Skinner TM, Gross MT 2003 Limb length inequality: clinical implications for assessment and intervention. Journal of Orthopaedics and Sports Physical Therapy 33(5):221–234

Gurney B 2002 Leg length discrepancy. Gait and Posture 15(2):195–206

Harris I, Hatfield A, Walton J 2005 Assessing leg length discrepancy after femoral fracture: clinical examination or computed tomography? Australia and New Zealand Journal of Surgery 75(5):319–321

Mannello DM 1992 Leg length inequality. Journal of Manipulative and Physiological Therapeutics 15(9):576–587

Middleton-Duff T, George K, Batterham A 2000 The reliability and validity of the 'tape' and 'block' methods for assessing anatomical leg-length discrepancy. Physical Therapy in Sport 1(3):91–99

Table A.4

Tape measure: spinal movements

Study	Aim of study	Numbers	Methodology	Results
Gauvin et al (1990)	To assess the intra-therapist (intrarater) and inter-therapist (interrater) reliability of measurements of forward bending with the modified fingertip-to-floor (MFTF) method on patients with low back pain (LBP)	73 patients with LBP participated in the study. Six physical therapists were randomly allocated to take the measurements	Each patient stood on a stool 32.4 cm high and bent forwards. The clinician measured, with a tape measure, from the tip of the middle finger to the top of the stool. An investigator recorded the reading. The clinician then took a second measurement, which was again recorded by an investigator. A second clinician then took two measurements of the same patient, recorded by the same investigator	The intraclass correlation coefficient (ICC) was calculated to assess the inter- and intratester reliability. The ICC for intratester reliability was calculated by comparing the first and second measurements taken by all the clinicians (146 in total). The ICC for intertester reliability was calculated by comparing the first measurements taken by the two clinicians. The ICC for intratester reliability was 0.98 and for intertester reliability was 0.95. The authors concluded that the MFTF method appears to be a very reliable method for measuring forward bending of patients with LBP. They also said that further research was required to determine the criterion validity

(table continues)

Table A.4 (continued)

Study	Aim of study	Numbers	Methodology	Results
Haywood et al (2004)	To examine the measurement properties of this evidence-based selection of spinal mobility measures in ankylosing spondylitis (AS) patients	159 patients with ankylosing spondylitis participated in the study	The measurements assessed were as follows: cervical rotation (Crot); finger-to-floor distance (FFD); lumbar lateral flexion (LLF); modified Schober index (MSI); tragus-to-wall distance (TWD) All the measurement were taken using a tape measure For the assessment of interobserver reliability, two observers recorded the baseline measurements for all the participants, following a randomized order of assessment For the assessment of intraobserver reliability, one observer repeated the measurements at 2 weeks The participants also completed a health transition questionnaire	Reliability estimates support the use of all measures in individual evaluation, where the intraclass correlation coefficients (ICCs) were >0.90 The authors conclude that they would recommend the use of MSI, Crot and FFD as reflecting spinal mobility in AS. They state that the measures are inexpensive and simple to administer in clinical practice and have evidence for reliability and validity
Jordan (2000)	To assess the reliability of tools to measure cervical spine range of motion (ROM) in clinical settings		This paper is a systematic review of the tools to measure ROM of the cervical spine. The author reviews 21 papers, which are presented in table form	

Viitanen et al (1998)	To assess clinically different cervical ranges of motion, including two new measurements of cervical lateral flexion and rotation, using a tape measure method compared with measurements using the Myrin inclinometer technique	52 male patients with ankylosing spondylitis (AS) participated in the study	The examiner measured the distance between the ear lobe (tragus) and the (tuberculum) coronoideus claviculae with a tape measure from the zero position (head erect) to maximal bending on both sides (right and left) without rotation for assessment of cervical lateral flexion

They also measured the distance between the top of the chin and the coronoideus claviculae with a tape measure from the zero position (chin straight ahead) to maximal rotation on both sides

Repeated tests were measured twice on successive days by one examiner for intratester reliability and a second examiner for interobserver reliability | All measurements showed good reliability, intraclass correlation coefficients (ICCs) ranged from 0.89 to 0.98

The authors conclude that the two new tape methods for measuring cervical rotation and lateral bending were as valid and reliable as the inclinometer method, but also quick and easy |

REFERENCES

Gauvin MG, Riddle DL, Rothstein JM 1990 Reliability of clinical measurements of forward bending using the modified fingertip-to-floor method. Physical Therapy 70(7):443–447

Haywood KL, Garratt AM, Jordan K, Dziedzic K, Dawes PT 2004 Spinal mobility in ankylosing spondylitis: reliability, validity and responsiveness. Rheumatology 43(6):750–757

Jordan K 2000 Assessment of published reliability studies for cervical spine range-of-motion measurement tools. Journal of Manipulative and Physiological Therapeutics 23(3):180–195

Viitanen JV, Kokko M-L, Heikkilä S, Kautiainen H 1998 Neck mobility assessment in ankylosing spondylitis: a clinical study of nine measurements including new tape methods for cervical rotation and lateral flexion. British Journal of Rheumatology 37(4):377–381

Table A.5

Tape measure: chest expansion

Study	Aim of study	Numbers	Methodology	Results
Bockenhauer et al (2007)	To assess the reliability of measuring thoracic excursion at two levels with a tape measure	Six healthy male subjects participated in the study. Five subjects participated in session 1 and four subjects participated in session 2. Three examiners took the measurements	Upper thoracic excursion was measured at the level of the 5th thoracic spinous process and the 3rd intercostal space, at the mid-clavicular level. The lower thoracic excursion was measured at the level of the 10th thoracic spinous process and the xiphoid process. Measurements of thoracic excursion were taken in two sessions. In session 1, five subjects were measured and interexaminer reliability was enhanced by asking the subject to hold their breath during the inhalation and exhalation while the three examiners took measurements successively. In session 2, four subjects were measured separately by the three examiners, thus allowing a full respiratory cycle to be measured by each examiner	The intraclass correlation coefficients (ICCs) ranged from 0.81 to 0.91 at both measurements in both sessions. When inhalation and exhalation were considered separately, interexaminer ICCs were 0.99 or greater. The authors conclude that the study strongly suggests that the tape measure method of measuring thoracic excursion at two levels could be reliable and useful in a clinical setting

(table continues)

Table A.5 (continued)

Study	Aim of study	Numbers	Methodology	Results
Custers et al (2005)	To determine the reliability of thoracic excursion measurement (TEM) and its relation to pulmonary function and height in children with cystic fibrosis (CF)	30 children and adolescents with CF participated in the intraobserver reliability study 30 other children and adolescents with CF participated in the interobserver reliability study	The subjects were positioned in supine lying. The tape measure was set around the chest at the axillary level. The subjects were asked to inhale and exhale calmly and the thoracic circumference was measured. The subjects were then asked to inhale and exhale maximally and measurements were taken at maximum inhalation and expiration The same procedure was repeated at the xiphoid level For the intraobserver reliability study one observer performed two consecutive measurements on each subject For the interobserver reliability study two observers performed a single measurement independently, on another patient group of 30 subjects, using the same protocol as previously	There was a negligible difference between the means of the thoracic excursion measurement (TEM) in the intraobserver reliability study, and the typical error was 0.31 cm Comparing the results from tester 1 and tester 2 in the interobserver reliability study revealed a mean difference of 0.12 cm, with a typical error of 0.56 cm TEM correlated significantly with height Thoracic excursion was moderately correlated with pulmonary function The authors conclude that thoracic excursion measurement (TEM) on children with CF is reliable, simple and takes little time

| Sharma et al (2004) | To examine the intra-tester reliability and intertester reliability of chest expansion (CE) using a tape measure, in subjects with ankylosing spondylitis (AS) and healthy subjects | 22 subjects with ankylosing spondylitis and 25 healthy subjects participated in the study. The AS patients were measured on two occasions by three investigators. The healthy subjects were measured on two occasions by two investigators | The measurement of each subject was taken at the level of the xiphisternum in standing, using two different arm positions: hands on head and arms at the side. Measurements of CE were taken using a tape measure. The tester measured the difference between maximal inspiration and maximal expiration. Each investigator took three trials in each position. There was a 10-minute break between taking the first and second sets of measurements | The intraclass correlation coefficients (ICCs) for intratester reliability for the AS subjects ranged from 0.85 to 0.97 and for the healthy subjects ranged from 0.90 to 0.96. The intertester reliability using the ICC was found to be very high in both groups in both arm positions. The ICC for the hand to head position in the AS group was 0.97 and arms to sides was 0.96. The ICC for the healthy subject group for the hands to head position was 0.95 and arms to sides was 0.93 |

REFERENCES

Bockenhauer S, Chen H, Julliard KN, Weedon J 2007 Measuring thoracic excursion: reliability of the cloth tape measure technique. Journal of American Osteopathic Association 107(5):191–196

Custers JWH, Arets HGM, Engelbert RHH, Kooijmans FTC, van der Ent CK, Helders PJM 2005 Thoracic excursion measurement in children with cystic fibrosis. Journal of Cystic Fibrosis 4(2):129–133

Sharma J, Senjyu H, Williams L, White C 2004 Intra-tester and inter-tester reliability of chest expansion measurement in clients with ankylosing spondylitis and healthy individuals. Journal of the Japanese Physical Therapy Association 7(1):23–28

Studies assessing reliability and validity

Table A.6

Grip strength

Study	Aim of study	Numbers	Methodology	Results
Bohannon et al (2006)	The purpose of the meta-analysis was to consolidate the results of studies presenting normative values for grip strength obtained with the Jamar dynamometer in accordance with the recommendations of the American Society of Hand Therapists (ASHT)	12 studies (3317 subjects) were identified and reviewed by the authors	The authors performed an extensive search of the literature from 1982 to 2004. Key words were: hand, grip, strength, dynamometer, Jamar, norms, and reference values	The study presents age-, gender- and side-specific reference values for hand grip strength derived from a meta-analysis of multinational data. The authors conclude that the norms can be used in lieu of more limited data previously available from individual studies
Coldham et al (2006)	To establish the test–retest reliability of taking one and three maximal isometric grip strength readings in symptomatic and asymptomatic subjects. To compare the test–retest reliability of one versus the mean of three trials and the highest of three trials in symptomatic and asymptomatic subjects	66 subjects participated in the study. 22 subjects were asymptomatic, 22 were post carpal tunnel decompression and 22 were post flexor tendon repair	Pre- and post-testing pain levels were recorded using a verbal analogue scale, where 0 equals no pain and 10 the worst pain imaginable. Grip strength testing was performed on a Jamar dynamometer using a standard testing protocol advocated by the American Society of Hand Therapists (ASHT). Half of the subjects were randomly selected to perform three trials followed by	All the three methods of grip strength measurement (one trial, the mean of three trials, and the highest of three trials) demonstrated high levels of test–retest reliability with ICCs of ≥0.85. A significant difference ($P = 0.0001$) was observed in all three subject groups between the highest of the three trials and the mean of the three trials. Clinically acceptable levels of reliability (≥0.91) were demonstrated by all three methods of grip strength testing other

(table continues)

Table A.6 (continued)

Study	Aim of study	Numbers	Methodology	Results
	To evaluate the level of pain experienced by subjects during the grip test		one, with the other half performing one trial followed by the three After a sufficient rest period the entire protocol was repeated. If the subject had completed three trials followed by one they would now perform one trial followed by the three and vice versa	than the mean of the three trials for the asymptomatic group A significant difference ($P = 0.0001$) was found in the reported pain levels after one trial and after three trials in each group The authors conclude that the findings of the study indicate that performing one grip strength trial is as reliable and less painful to perform than either the best of or the mean of three trials
Massy-Westropp et al (2004)	To determine age- and gender-specific reference values for the Grippit electronic dynamometer, and to compare measurements obtained from the two instruments (Jamar dynamometer and Grippit electronic dynamometer)	419 healthy subjects participated in the study. Subjects were divided according to age and gender Each subject performed a grip strength test on each hand, using both instruments	Grip strength testing was performed on a Jamar dynamometer using a standard testing protocol advocated by the American Society of Hand Therapists (ASHT). Grip strength was tested on the Grippit dynamometer according to the manufacturer's instructions, with a 10-second measurement period Participants chose which hand and which instrument they used first	Age- and gender-specific reference ranges for grip strength measured with the Jamar and Grippit dynamometers are presented Grip strength peaks in the third and fourth decade of life for both men and women The authors conclude that both instruments were easy to use, although there were difficulties in standardising the positioning of some subjects when using the table-mounted Grippit dynamometer They also said the Grippit can detect the low grip strength scores that cannot be detected by the Jamar

Mathiowetz (2002)	To compare the Jamar and Rolyan hydraulic dynamometers to determine their concurrent validity with known weights as well as their inter-instrument reliability and concurrent validity for measuring grip strength in a clinical setting	A convenience sample of 30 healthy males and 30 healthy females participated in the study	The concurrent validity of the Jamar and Rolyan dynamometers with known weights (the relationship between the instrument readout and applied force) was evaluated before and after the study The subjects were seated with their shoulders adducted and neutrally rotated, elbow flexed at 90°, forearm in neutral and wrist between 0° and 30° of flexion and between 0° and 15° of ulnar deviation Each subject undertook three successive measurements for the right hand and for the left hand on the two dynamometers. The mean of the three trials was used for data analysis	Concurrent validity with known weights for the Jamar dynamometer was $r = 0.9998$ and 0.9998 (before and after the study) and for the Rolyan dynamometer was $r = 0.9994$ and 0.9997 (before and after the study) The intraclass correlation coefficients (ICCs) between the two dynamometers ranged from 0.90 to 0.97, which suggests excellent inter-instrument reliability

(table continues)

Table A.6 (continued)

Study	Aim of study	Numbers	Methodology	Results
Molenaar et al (2008)	To compare the reliability of a Jamar-like dynamometer with that of the Martin vigorimeter for measurement of the hand strength of children (4–12 years old)	104 primary school children participated in the study	The grip strength of both hands was measured with an electronic Jamar-like dynamometer and the Martin vigorimeter During the measurement with the Jamar-like dynamometer, all the children were seated and the testing protocol advocated by the American Society of Hand Therapists (ASHT) was used. The medium bulb was used for the Martin vigorimeter and the subject's forearm rested in neutral on the table with the wrist in 0° to 30° of extension The mean of three maximum voluntary contractions performed with each instrument was recorded for each hand The retest was performed under the same conditions after a mean interval of 29 days	In the total group, the intraclass correlation coefficient (ICC) for the Jamar-like dynamometer was 0.97 for the dominant hand and 0.95 for the non-dominant hand The intraclass correlation coefficient (ICC) for the Martin vigorimeter was 0.84 for the dominant hand and 0.86 for the non-dominant hand The authors conclude the data suggest that the Jamar-like dynamometer can more reliably measure the grip strength of children

Shechtman et al (2005)	To examine the reliability and validity of the DynEx digital dynamometer and compare it with the criterion standard, hydraulic, Jamar dynamometer for measurement of maximal hand grip strength among healthy subjects	100 healthy subjects participated in the study	The calibration of the dynamometers was verified using known weights suspended from the dynamometer's handle The subjects were seated with their shoulders adducted and neutrally rotated, elbow flexed at 90°, forearm in neutral and wrist between 0° and 30° of flexion and between 0° and 15° of ulnar deviation Each subject performed two sessions of grip strength testing, one on the Jamar dynamometer and one on the DynEx dynamometer. Each test consisted of three maximal repeated contractions, gripping first with the right hand and then the left hand After a 10-minute break the entire protocol was repeated for a total of 12 grip repetitions per hand	The DynEx dynamometer was found to have high test–retest reliability both with human subjects (r = 0.9864) and with known weights (r = 0.9999) The concurrent validity between the two dynamometers was excellent (r > 0.98)

REFERENCES

Bohannon RW, Peolsson A, Massy-Westropp N, Desrosiers J, Bear-Lehman J 2006 Reference values for adult grip strength measured with a Jamar dynamometer: a descriptive meta-analysis. Physiotherapy 92(1):11–15

Coldham F, Lewis J, Lee H 2006 The reliability of one vs three grip trials in symptomatic and asymptomatic subjects. Journal of Hand Therapy 19(3):318–327

Massy-Westropp N, Rankin W, Ahern M, Krishnan J, Hearn TC 2004 Measuring grip strength in normal adults: reference ranges and a comparison of electronic and hydraulic instruments. Journal of Hand Surgery 29A(3):514–519

Mathiowetz V 2002 Comparison of Rolyan and Jamar dynamometers for measuring grip strength. Occupational Therapy International 9(3):201–209

Molenaar HM, Zuidam JM, Selles RW, Stam HJ, Hovius SER 2008 Age-specific reliability of two grip-strength dynamometers when used by children. Journal of Bone and Joint Surgery American 90:1053–1059

Shechtman O, Gestewitz L, Kimble C 2005 Reliability and validity of the DynEx dynamometer. Journal of Hand Therapy 18(3):339–347

Studies assessing reliability and validity

Table A.7

Muscle strength

Study	Aim of study	Numbers	Methodology	Results
Bø & Finckenhagen (2001)	To evaluate the intertester reproducibility of the modified Oxford grading system for vaginal palpation, and to compare results from vaginal palpation with vaginal squeeze pressure	20 female students participated in the study. Two experienced therapists conducted the study	Each subject was taught how to contract their pelvic floor muscles (PFMs). On contracting their PFMs the first therapist performed a vaginal palpation, firstly by classifying the contraction in a qualitative way (no contraction; contraction; contraction with help of other muscles; uncertain and straining). They then graded the contraction according to the modified Oxford grading system (0 = no contraction; 1 = flicker; 2 = weak; 3 = moderate; 4 = good; 5 = strong). After a 5-minute rest the procedure was repeated by the second therapist. The PFM strength was then measured by vaginal squeeze pressure	Based on the qualitative classification, the two therapists classified 19 of the participants to have performed correct PFM contractions. The interrater reliability for vaginal palpation was 0.70 measured by Spearman's rho ($P < 0.01$). The authors conclude the present results indicate that this method is not reproducible, sensitive and valid to measure PFM strength for scientific purposes
Bø & Sherburn (2005)	To give an overview of evaluation methods available to measure pelvic floor muscle (PFM) function and strength and to discuss the advantages and disadvantages of the different methods			

(table continues)

Table A.7 (continued)

Study	Aim of study	Numbers	Methodology	Results
Bohannon (2005)	To evaluate the adequacy of manual muscle testing as a screening test relative to dynamometry	A convenience sample of 107 elderly patients, presenting with a variety of diagnoses	Manual muscle testing, maximum voluntary knee extension, was measured bilaterally using manual muscle testing (MMT) and a hand-held dynamometer	The author concludes that the study casts doubt on the suitability of manual muscle testing as a screening test for strength impairment
Cuthbert & Goodheart (2007)	The aim of this review is to provide an historical overview, literature review, description, synthesis and critique of the reliability and validity of manual muscle testing (MMT) in the evaluation of the musculoskeletal and nervous systems	Over 100 studies were found and reviewed by the authors	The authors performed an extensive search of the literature from 1915 to 2006. Key words were: manual muscle testing, manual muscle test, and applied kinesiology. Over 100 articles were found and reviewed by the authors. 12 studies were randomized controlled trials (RCTs)	The authors conclude that MMT employed by chiropractics, therapists and neurologists was shown to be a clinically useful tool
Escolar et al (2001)	To compare the reliability of 12 clinical evaluators in performing manual muscle testing (MMT) and quantitative muscle testing (QMT) on 12 children with muscular dystrophy	12 ambulatory children with neuromuscular disease participated in the study. 12 experienced evaluators performed the testing	The children were scored by the modified Medical Research Council scale on five muscle groups, bilaterally (shoulder abductors, elbow flexors, hip flexors, knee extensors and ankle dorsiflexors). Quantitative muscle testing (QMT) was then performed bilaterally on four muscle groups (grip, knee extensors, ankle dorsiflexors and elbow flexors) by recording the maximal voluntary isometric contraction (MVIC)	Quantitative muscle testing (QMT) was reliable, with an intraclass correlation coefficient (ICC) of >0.9 for elbow flexors and grip strength, and >0.8 for the knee extensors. Manual muscle testing (MMT) was not as reliable and required repeated training for evaluators to achieve an ICC >0.75 for shoulder

		All the subjects were tested four times over a 2-day period

The interrater consistency of examinations was assessed by comparing three groups of four clinical evaluators testing the same four subjects each

A second reliability study for MMT was performed 2 months later using two groups of evaluators | abductors, elbow and hip flexors, knee extensors and ankle dorsiflexors

The authors conclude that QMT shows greater reliability and is easier to implement than MMT |
| Florence et al (1992) | To evaluate the intrarater reliability of manual muscle test (MMT) grades in assessing muscle strength in patients with Duchenne's muscular dystrophy (DMD) | 102 boys with a diagnosis of DMD participated in the study. All the subjects were required to perform the MMT

Four experienced physical therapists undertook the examinations | Data were collected as part of a 12-month trial to document the effects of prednisone on muscle strength in patients with DMD. Two identical assessments were performed within 5 days of each other initially and after 6 and 12 months of treatment. Muscle strength was assessed and individual MMT grades were assigned using a modified Medical Research Council grading scale

18 muscle groups were assessed in each subject at each session | Intrarater reliability ranged from 0.65 to 0.93, with the proximal muscles having the higher reliability values

The authors conclude that the manual muscle test grades are reliable for assessing muscle strength in boys with DMD when consecutive evaluations are performed by the same physical therapist |

(table continues)

Table A.7 (continued)

Study	Aim of study	Numbers	Methodology	Results
Great Lakes ALS Study Group (2003)	To assess the reliability of strength testing techniques among centres investigating patients with amyotrophic lateral sclerosis (ALS). The strength tests performed were the manual muscle testing (MMT) and maximal voluntary isometric contraction (MVIC)	63 patients with ALS enrolled on the study, but only 48 patients completed the study	All subjects underwent two examinations by two different examiners within a week of enrolling on the study. MMT and MVIC testing was undertaken at each session. The MMT was derived from the Medical Research Council scale, where each muscle is scored from 0 to 5. In total, 34 muscles were tested. MVIC was measured in six muscle groups. At 6 months, two examiners each examined the subjects twice	Both techniques, when performed by trained therapists, were highly and equally reproducible. MMT was more sensitive than MVIC in detecting change over time in these patients. The authors conclude the findings of the study demonstrate that MMT performed by experienced therapists is a reliable and reproducible method of assessing disease progression in ALS

REFERENCES

Bø K and Finckenhagen HB 2001 Vaginal palpation of pelvic floor muscle strength: inter-test reproducibility and comparison between palpation and vaginal squeeze pressure. Acta Obstetrica et Gynecologica Scandinavica 80(10):883–887

Bø K and Sherburn M 2005 Evaluation of female pelvic-floor muscle function and strength. Physical Therapy 85(3):269–282

Bohannon RW 2005 Manual muscle testing: does it meet the standards of an adequate screening test? Clinical Rehabilitation 19(6):662–667

Cuthbert SC and Goodheart GJ 2007 On the reliability and validity of manual muscle testing: a literature review. Chiropractic and Osteopathy 15:4

Escolar DM, Henricson EK, Mayhew J et al 2001 Clinical evaluator reliability for quantitative and manual muscle testing measures of strength in children. Muscle and Nerve 24(6):787–793

Florence JM, Pandya S, King WM et al 1992 Intrarater reliability of manual muscle test (Medical Research Council scale) grades in Duchenne's muscular dystrophy. Physical Therapy 72(2):115–126

Great Lakes ALS Study Group 2003 A comparison of muscle strength testing techniques in amyotrophic lateral sclerosis. Neurology 61:1503–1507

Medical Research Council (MRC) 1976 Aids to the investigation of the peripheral nervous system. London: Her Majesty's Stationery Office

Table A.8

Spirometry

Study	Aim of study	Numbers	Methodology	Results
Crapo & Jensen (2003)	This is a very interesting symposium paper that discusses the standards and interpretive issues in lung function testing		The paper discusses the following issues: 1. Standards for lung function testing: what do they do? 2. What can you do? 3. Lung function testing: interpretive issues for doctors and respiratory therapists 4. Summary	
Enright (2003)	This is an interesting and informative paper that seeks to make sure your spirometry tests are of good quality			
Koyama et al (1998)	To compare four types of portable peak flow meters (PFMs) (Mini-Wright, Assess, Pulmo-graph and Wright Pocket meters) against spirometric peak expiratory flow rate (PEFR) and evaluate the agreement of the reading between each PFM	127 patients with chronic obstructive pulmonary disease (COPD), 120 patients with asthma, 34 patients with diffuse panbronchiolitis and 15 patients with other respiratory	Initially, spirometry was performed, in the standing position, by each subject, until three acceptable forced expiratory curves were obtained. After resting for 3–4 min, each subject, in a standing position, blew into the Mini-Wright, Assess, Pulmo-graph and Wright Pocket meters three times in random order	The results of the study demonstrated that the readings of all four types of standard range PFMs had an equivalent correlation coefficient with spirometric PEFRs, indicating that each

Studies assessing reliability and validity

	symptoms and 15 healthy volunteers participated in the study	The highest value of the three blows was recorded in each PFM measurement Finally, a second series of spirometric measures was performed, in the standing position, by each subject, until three acceptable forced expiratory curves were obtained. The second spirometric PEFR was used as a standard against which the reading of the PFM was compared	PFM gave a similarly valid reading when a spirometric PEFR was taken as a representative of the true value The authors conclude that all four types of the standard range PFMs have an equivalent validity
Miller et al (2005a)	This document brings the views of the American Thoracic Society (ATS) and the European Respiratory Society (ERS) together in an attempt to publish guidelines on the standardization of lung function testing. This document contains details about procedures that are common for many methods of lung function testing		
Miller et al (2005b)	This document brings the views of the American Thoracic Society (ATS) and the European Respiratory Society (ERS) together in an attempt to publish guidelines on the standardization of lung function testing This document contains details about the standardization of spirometry		

(table continues)

Table A.8 (continued)

Study	Aim of study	Numbers	Methodology	Results
Pellegrino et al (2005)	This document brings the views of the American Thoracic Society (ATS) and the European Respiratory Society (ERS) together in an attempt to publish guidelines on the standardization of lung function testing This document contains details to provide guidance in interpreting pulmonary function tests			
White (2004)	This is an interesting paper, which considers the factors that limit the use of spirometry in routine primary care consultations and makes a proposal for the integration of peak expiratory flow (PEF) and spirometry in the objective assessment of chronic obstructive pulmonary disease (COPD) outcome		The author concludes that spirometry is essential in the diagnosis of COPD, but as the decline in lung function is slow, spirometry is unlikely to provide significantly new information more than every 1–2 years. The author suggests that there is no evidence that in a patient already diagnosed with COPD spirometry provides more information than PEF in the day-to-day management of the condition	

REFERENCES

Crapo RO, Jensen RL 2003 Standards and interpretive issues in lung function testing. Respiratory Care 48(8):764–772

Enright PL 2003 How to make sure your spirometry tests are of good quality. Respiratory Care 48(8):773–776

Koyama H, Nishimura K, Ikeda A, Tsukino M, Izumi T 1998 Comparison of four types of portable peak flow meters (Mini-Wright, Assess, Pulmo-graph and Wright Pocket meters). Respiratory Medicine 92(3):505–511

Miller MR, Crapo R, Hankinson J et al 2005a General considerations for lung function testing. European Respiratory Journal 26:153–161

Miller MR, Hankinson J, Brusasco V et al 2005b Standardisation of spirometry. European Respiratory Journal 26:319–338

Pellegrino R, Viegi G, Brusasco V et al 2005 Interpretive strategies for lung function tests. European Respiratory Journal 26(5):948–968

White P 2004 Spirometry and peak expiratory flow in the primary care management of COPD. Primary Care Respiratory Journal 13(1):5–8

Table A.9

Visual analogue scale (VAS) and the numeric rating scale (NRS)

Study	Aim of study	Numbers	Methodology	Results
Gallagher et al (2002)	To assess the reliability and validity of the visual analogue scale (VAS) in the measurement of acute abdominal pain in the emergency department (ED)	101 patients with acute abdominal pain were enrolled in the study	Patients were asked to rate their abdominal pain severity by placing a vertical mark on a 100 mm horizontal VAS. The left and right extremes of the VAS were labelled 'least possible pain' and 'worst possible pain', respectively. One minute later the patients were again asked to rate their pain severity, without reference to the first measurement. This procedure was repeated every 30 minutes for 2 hours. After completing the VAS at the end of each 30-minute interval, the patients were also asked to contrast current pain with their pain at the time of the previous measurement, using one of five categorical descriptors: 'much less pain', 'a little less pain', 'about the same pain', 'a little more pain', or 'much more pain'	Reliability was high, with the intraclass correlation coefficient (ICC) between VAS scores 1 minute apart being 0.99. To assess validity, the mean and median VAS change scores increased linearly and in a graduated fashion as the pain descriptors escalated from 'much less pain' to 'much more pain'. The authors conclude that the VAS is a reliable and valid instrument for measuring acute abdominal pain in the ED

Litcher-Kelly et al (2007)	To search the literature for the year 2003 and to investigate which pain assessments are most commonly used in clinical trials	Articles addressing chronic musculoskeletal pain in clinical trials were identified in seven major medical journals for the year 2003; 50 studies met the selection criteria	The authors performed an extensive search of the literature for the year 2003 in seven major medical journals. 50 studies were selected for review, 66% were randomized controlled trials (RCTs) and 34% were controlled trials	The most frequently used assessments were the single-item visual analogue scale (VAS) and the numeric rating scale (NRS). The authors conclude that overall, it appears that clinical trials use simple measures of pain
Lundeberg et al (2001)	To evaluate the intra-individual disagreement in assessments of pain made independently with the visual analogue scale (VAS), the numeric rating scale (NRS) and the painmatcher	69 patients with chronic neurogenic pain participated in the study	The patients were asked to rate their intensity of pain using the VAS, NRS and the painmatcher. The whole assessment procedure was repeated. The patients were then treated with transcutaneous electrical nerve stimulation (TENS) for 30 minutes. At the end of treatment, pain levels were again assessed using the same procedures as before	The results of the study show that the painmatcher and ratings of perceived pain using VAS and NRS all have a comparable reliability with acceptable stability in determining the perceived intensity of pain and assessing pain-controlling interventions for the group

REFERENCES

Gallagher EJ, Bijur PE, Latimer C, Silver W 2002 Reliability and validity of a visual analog scale for acute abdominal pain in the ED (Emergency Department). American Journal of Emergency Medicine 20(4):287–290

Litcher-Kelly L, Martino SA, Broderick JE, Stone AA 2007 A systematic review of measures used to assess chronic musculoskeletal pain in clinical and randomized controlled clinical trials. Journal of Pain 8(12):906–913

Lundeberg T, Lund I, Dahlin L et al 2001 Reliability and responsiveness of three different pain assessments. Journal of Rehabilitation and Medicine 33(6):279–283

Index

A

Abductor pollicis brevis, 175
Abductor pollicis longus, 175
Adductor brevis, 6
Adductor longus, 6
Adductor magnus, 6
Anconeus, 128
Ankle joint, 59–87
  anatomy, 59–64
  bony landmarks, 59–60
  calf girth, 75–6
  joint girth, 72–4
  ligaments, 60
  limb girth, 75–6
  muscles, 61–4
    dorsiflexors, 62
    evertors, 64
    invertors, 63
    plantarflexors, 61
  muscle strength: Oxford muscle grading, 77–87
    dorsiflexors, 79–81
    evertors, 82–3
    invertors, 84–6
    notes, 87
    plantarflexors, 77–9
    treatment record, 87
  range of movement, 65–71
    dorsiflexion, 65
    eversion, 69
    inversion, 67–8
    notes, 70
    observational/reflective checklist, 71
    plantarflexion, 66
    treatment record, 70
Annular ligament, 126
Anterior cruciate ligament, 42
Anterior ligament (ankle), 60
Anterior longitudinal ligament, 188
Anterior oblique ligament, 174
Anterior radiate ligament, 211
Anterior superior iliac spine (ASIS), 2
Anterior talofibular ligament, 60
Anterior tibiotalar band, 60
Arm girth, 104–6

B

Biceps brachii, long head, 91, 127, 129
Biceps femoris, 3, 44, 46
Brachialis, 127
Brachioradialis, 127, 129, 130

C

Calcaneofibular ligament, 60
Calf
  girth, 75–6
  muscle bulk, 50
Capitate, 174
Carpal joint *see* Wrist/carpal joints
Carpometacarpal (CMC) joint of the thumb, 173, 176–7
  abduction, 176–7
  flexion/extension, 177
  see also Hand; Wrist/carpal joints
Carpus, 150, 174
Cervical measurement system, x
Cervical spine *see* Neck

Chest expansion
  measurement, 213–15
    studies assessing the reliability of tape measures, 243–5
Compass goniometer, 207
Construct validity, ix
Content validity, ix
Coracoacromial ligament, 90
Coracobrachialis, 91, 93
Coracohumeral ligament, 90
Coronary ligaments, 42
Costochondral joint, 211
Costotransverse joint, 212
Costotransverse ligament, 212
Costovertebral joint, 212
Criterion validity, x

D

Deltoid, 91, 92, 94, 95
Deltoid ligament, 60
Diaphragm, 210
Distal interphalangeal (DIP) joint of the finger, 174, 183
Dorsal radiocarpal ligament, 150
Dynamometer, 170–1, xi

E

Elbow joint, 125–48
  anatomy, 125–30
  bony landmarks, 126
  joint girth, 137–8
  ligaments, 126
  muscles, 127–30
    extensors, 128
    flexors, 127
    pronators, 130
    supinators, 129
  muscle strength: Oxford muscle grading, 139–48
    extensors, 139–41
    flexors, 141–3
    pronators, 146–8
    supinators, 144–6
  range of movement, 131–6
    extension, 132
    flexion, 131
    notes, 135
    observational/reflective checklist, 136
    pronation, 134
    supination, 133
    treatment record, 135
Erector spinae, 190, 192
Extensor carpi radialis brevis, 152, 153
Extensor carpi radialis longus, 152, 153
Extensor carpi ulnaris, 152, 154
Extensor digiti minimi, 152
Extensor digitorum, 152
Extensor digitorum longus, 62
Extensor hallucis longus, 62
Extensor indicis, 152
Extensor pollicis brevis, 153, 174
Extensor pollicis longus, 153, 174
External oblique, 189

F

Face validity, ix
Femur, 42
  greater trochanter, 2, 9
Fibula, 42, 60
Fingers
  distal interphalangeal joint, 174, 183
  metacarpophalangeal joint, 173
    abduction, 181
    flexion, 180
  proximal interphalangeal joint, 174, 182
Flexor carpi radialis, 151, 153
Flexor carpi ulnaris, 151, 154
Flexor digitorum longus, 61
Flexor digitorum profundus, 151
Flexor digitorum superficialis, 151
Flexor hallucis longus, 61
Flexor pollicis brevis, 175
Flexor pollicis longus, 151, 175
Foot, 60
Forced expiratory volume in one second (FEV_1), 216–17, xii
Forced vital capacity (FVC), 216–17, xii

G

Gastrocnemius, 44, 61
Gemellus inferior, 7
Gemellus superior, 7
Glenoid fossa, 90
Glenoid labrum, 90
Gluteus maximus, 3, 5, 7
Gluteus medius, 5, 8
Gluteus minimus, 5, 8
Goniometers
  compass, 207
  studies assessing reliability, 221–8
Goniometric measurement, x
Gracilis, 6, 44, 45
Greater trochanter of the femur, 2, 9
Grip
  Jamar hand dynamometer, xi
  strength, 170–1, 247–51

H

Hamate, 174
Hamstrings, 3
Hand, 173–85
  anatomy, 173–6
  bony landmarks, 174
  ligaments, 174
  muscles, 174–6
    abductors, 175–6
    adductors, 175–6
    extensors, 174
    flexors, 175
    opposers, 175–6
  range of movement, 176–85
    finger
      distal interphalangeal joint, 183
      metacarpophalangeal joint
        abduction, 181
        flexion, 180
      proximal interphalangeal joint, 182
    notes, 184
    observational/reflective checklist, 185
    thumb
      carpometacarpal joint, 176–7
        abduction, 176–7
        flexion/extension, 177
      interphalangeal joint, 179
      metacarpophalangeal joint, 178
    treatment record, 184
Hand-held dynamometer, 170–1, xi
Hip joint, 1–39
  anatomy, 1–8
  bony landmarks, 2
  leg length, 36–9
    apparent shortening, 36, 38
    true length of limb, 38
    true shortening, 36, 38
  ligaments, 2
  muscle bulk, 17–19
  muscles, 3–8
    abductors, 5
    adductors, 6
    extensors, 3
    flexors, 4
    lateral rotators, 7
    medial rotators, 8
  muscle strength: Oxford muscle grading, 20–35
    abductors, 25–7
    adductors, 27–9
    extensors, 20–2
    flexors, 22–4
    lateral rotators, 30–2
    medial rotators, 32–4
    notes, 35
    treatment record, 35
  range of movement, 8–16
    abduction, 11
    adduction, 12
    extension, 9
    flexion, 10
    lateral rotation, 13
    medial rotation, 14
    notes, 15
    observational/reflective checklist, 16
    treatment record, 15
Humerus, 89, 126

I

Iliac crest, 2
Iliacus, 4
Iliocostalis cervicis, 190

Iliocostalis lumborum, 190
Iliocostalis thoracis, 190
Iliofemoral ligament, 2
Iliopubic eminence, 2
Inclinometer, 200–3, 205
Inferior glenohumeral ligament, 90
Inferior radioulnar joint, 126
  see also Elbow joint
Infraspinatus, 90, 94
Innominate bone, 2
Interchondral joints, 211–12
Intercostals, 210
Internal oblique, 189
International Knee Documentation Committee (IKDC), x–xi
Interphalangeal (IP) joint
  of the finger, 174
  of the thumb, 179
Interspinous ligaments, 188
Intertester (interobserver) reliability, ix
Intratester (intraobserver) reliability, ix
Ischial tuberosity, 2
Ischiofemoral ligament, 2

J

Jamar hand dynamometer, xi

K

Knee, 41–58
  anatomy, 41–6
  bony landmarks, 42
  joint girth, 48–9
  ligaments, 42
  muscle bulk, 49–51
    calf, 50
    thigh, 49–50
  muscles, 43–6
    extensors, 43
    flexors, 44
    lateral (external) rotators, 46
    medial (internal) rotators, 45
  muscle strength: Oxford muscle grading, 53–8
    extensors, 53–5
    flexors, 55–7
    notes, 58
    treatment record, 58
  range of movement, 46–8
    extension, 46–7, x–xi
    flexion, 47–8, x–xi
    hyperextension, x–xi
    notes, 52
    observational/reflective checklist, 52

L

Lateral collateral ligament, 42
Lateral costotransverse ligament, 212
Lateral ligament (ankle), 60
Latissimus dorsi, 92, 93, 95
Leg length, 36–9
  apparent shortening, 36, 38
  studies assessing the reliability of tape measures, 234–7
  true length of limb, 38
  true shortening, 36, 38
Ligamentum flavum, 188
Ligamentum nuchae, 188
Ligamentum teres, 2
Longissimus capitis, 190, 192
Longissimus cervicis, 190
Longissimus thoracis, 190
Lumbar spine
  extension, 193–4
  flexion, 192–3
  flexion/extension, 194–5
Lunate, 174

M

Manual muscle testing/Oxford grading, xi
  see also specific joint
Manubriosternal joint, 210
Medial collateral ligament, 42
Metacarpals, 174
Metacarpophalangeal (MCP) joint, 173
  finger
    abduction, 181
    flexion, 180
  thumb, 178

Index

Middle glenohumeral ligament, 90
Multifidus, 191
Muscle strength studies, 253–6

N

Neck
  extension, 202–3
  flexion, 199–201
    using an inclinometer, 200–1
    using a tape measure, 199
  lateral flexion, 204–5
    using an inclinometer, 205
    using a tape measure, 204
  muscles, 191–2
    extensors, 192
    flexors, 191
  range of motion, x
  rotation, 206–7
    using a compass goniometer, 207
    using a tape measure, 206
Numeric rating scale (NRS), 219, 262–3

O

Obturator internus, 7
Opponens pollicis, 176
Oxford grading, xi
  see also specific joint

P

Pain measurement, 219, 262–3
Palmaris brevis, 176
Palmaris longus, 151
Palmar radiocarpal ligament, 150
Palmar ulnocarpal ligament, 150
Patella, 42
Peak expiratory flow rate (PEFR), 218, xiv
Peak flow meter (PFM), xiv
Pectineus, 4, 6
Pectoralis major, 91, 92, 93, 95
Peroneus brevis, 64
Peroneus longus, 64
Peroneus tertius, 62, 64
Phalanges (hand), 174

Piriformis, 7
Pisiform, 174
Plantaris, 61
Popliteus, 45
Posterior cruciate ligament, 42
Posterior ligament (ankle), 60
Posterior longitudinal ligament, 188
Posterior oblique ligament, 174
Posterior radiate ligament, 211
Posterior superior iliac spine (PSIS), 2
Posterior talofibular ligament, 60
Posterior tibiotalar band, 60
Pronator quadratus, 130
Pronator teres, 127, 130
Proximal interphalangeal (PIP) joint of the finger, 174, 182
Psoas major, 4
Pubofemoral ligament, 2

Q

Quadrate ligament, 126
Quadratus lumborum, 191
Quadriceps girth measurement, 17

R

Radial carpometacarpal ligament, 174
Radial collateral ligament, 126, 150
Radiate ligament of the head of the rib, 213
Radiocarpal joint *see* Wrist/carpal joints
Radioulnar joint, 125–6
  see also Elbow joint
Radius, 126, 150
Range of motion (ROM), x
  see also specific joint
Rectus abdominis, 189
Rectus femoris, 4, 43
Reliability, ix
Respiratory system, 209–18
  anatomy, 209–13
  bony landmarks, 209
  chest expansion, 213–15
  joints of the thorax, 210–13
  ligaments, 211, 212, 213
  muscles, 210
  respiratory function, 216–18

Respiratory system (*continued*)
   FEV$_1$ and FVC, 216–17
   PEFR, 218
Rotator cuff muscles, 90
   see also specific muscles

S

Sartorious, 4, 44, 45
Scalenus anterior, 191
Scaphoid, 174
Scapula, 90
Schober test, modified, 194–5
Semimembranosus, 3, 44, 45
Semitendinosus, 3, 44, 45
Shoulder joint, 89–123
   anatomy, 89–95
   bony landmarks, 90
   ligaments, 90
   limb girth, 104–6
   muscles, 91–5
      abductors, 94
      adductors, 93
      extensors, 92
      flexors, 91
      lateral (external) rotators, 94
      medial (internal) rotators, 95
   muscle strength: Oxford muscle
         grading, 107–23
      abductors, 112–14
      adductors, 114–16
      extensors, 109–11
      flexors, 107–9
      lateral (external) rotators, 120–2
      medial (internal) rotators,
            117–20
      notes, 123
      treatment record, 123
   range of movement, 96–103
      abduction, 98
      adduction, 99
      extension, 96
      flexion, 97
      lateral (external) rotation, 101
      medial (internal) rotation, 100
      notes, 102
      observational/reflective checklist,
            103
      treatment record, 102
Soleus, 61

Spinalis capitis, 190
Spinalis cervicis, 190
Spinalis thoracis, 190
Spine, 187–207
   anatomy, 187–92
   bony landmarks, 197
   ligaments, 188
   muscles, 189–92
      neck flexors, 191
      trunk extensors, 190–1
      trunk flexors, 189
   range of movement, 192–207
      neck extension, 202–3
      neck flexion, 199–201
         using an inclinometer, 200–1
         using a tape measure, 199
      neck lateral flexion, 204–5
         using an inclinometer, 205
         using a tape measure, 204
      neck rotation, 206–7
         using a compass goniometer,
               207
         using a tape measure, 206
   notes, 197
   observational/reflective checklist,
         198
   studies assessing the reliability of
         tape measures, 239–41
   treatment record, 197
   trunk
      extension – lumbar spine,
            193–4
      flexion/extension – lumbar
            spine, 194–5
      flexion – lumbar spine, 192–3
      lateral (side) flexion, 196
Spinous processes, 197
Spirometry, xii–xv
   forced expiratory volume in one
         second (FEV$_1$), 216–17,
         xii
   forced vital capacity (FVC),
         216–17, xii
   peak expiratory flow rate (PEFR),
         218, xiv
   studies, 258–60
Splenius capitis, 192
Sternal joints, 210–11
Sternocostal joints, 211
Sternomastoid, 191
Subscapularis, 90, 95

Superior costotransverse ligament, 212
Superior glenohumeral ligament, 90
Superior radioulnar joint, 125–6
  see also Elbow joint
Supinator, 129
Supraspinatus, 90, 94
Supraspinous ligament, 188

T

Tape measure, xi
  studies assessing reliability
    chest expansion, 243–5
    leg length, 234–7
    limb/joint girth, 230–2
    spinal movements, 239–41
Tensor fascia lata, 4, 5, 8, 43
Teres major, 92, 93, 95
Teres minor, 90, 94
Thigh
  girth measurement, 17
  muscle bulk, 49–50
Thorax, joints of the, 210–13
Thumb
  carpometacarpal joint, 173, 176–7
    abduction, 176–7
    flexion/extension, 177
  interphalangeal joint, 179
  metacarpophalangeal joint, 178
Tibia, 42, 59
Tibialis anterior, 62, 63
Tibialis posterior, 61, 63
Tibiocalcaneal band, 60
Tibionavicular band, 60
Transverse humeral ligament, 90
Transverse ligament of the acetabulum, 2
Transversus abdominis, 189
Trapezium, 174
Trapezoid, 174
Triceps brachii, 92, 128
Triquetral, 174
Trunk
  extension – lumbar spine, 193–4
  flexion/extension – lumbar spine, 194
  flexion – lumbar spine, 192–3
  lateral (side) flexion, 196

U

Ulna, 126, 150
Ulnar collateral ligament, 126, 150
Upper limb girth, 104–6

V

Validity, ix–x
Vastus intermedius, 43
Vastus medialis, 43
Visual analogue pain scale (VAS), 219, 262–3
Vital capacity (VC), xii

W

Wrist/carpal joints, 149–71
  anatomy, 149–54
  bony landmarks, 150
  grip strength, 170–1
  joint girth, 169
  ligaments, 150
  muscles, 151–4
    abductors/radial deviators, 153
    adductors/ulnar deviators, 154
    extensors, 152–3
    flexors, 151
  muscle strength: Oxford muscle grading, 161–8
    abductors/radial deviators, 167–8
    adductors/ulnar deviators, 165–6
    extensors, 161–2
    flexors, 163–4
  range of movement, 155–60
    abduction/radial deviation, 158
    adduction/ulnar deviation, 157
    extension, 156
    flexion, 155
    notes, 159
    observational/reflective checklist, 160
    treatment record, 159

X

Xiphisternal joint, 211